Handbook of
Generalised Anxiety Disorder

Handbook of Generalised Anxiety Disorder

Stuart A Montgomery
Imperial College School of Medicine
London, UK

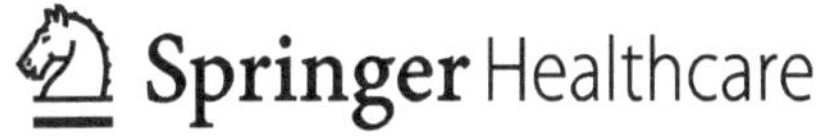

Published by Springer Healthcare, 236 Gray's Inn Road, London, WC1X 8HB, UK
www.currentmedicinegroup.com

Reprinted 2010

ISBN 978-1-85873-441-5

British Library Cataloguing-in-Publication Data.
A catalogue record for this book is available from the British Library.

Although every effort has been made to ensure that drug doses and other information are presented accurately in this publication, the ultimate responsibility rests with the prescribing physician. Neither the publisher nor the authors can be held responsible for errors or for any consequences arising from the use of the information contained herein. Any product mentioned in this publication should be used in accordance with the prescribing information prepared by the manufacturers. No claims or endorsements are made for any drug or compound at present under clinical investigation.

Commissioning editor: Ian Stoneham
Project editor: Lisa Langley
Designer: Joe Harvey and Taymoor Fouladi
Production: Marina Maher

Contents

Author biography

Dr Stuart A Montgomery is Emeritus Professor of Psychiatry at the Imperial College of Medicine in the University of London. He completed his undergraduate and postgraduate training in medicine at University College, University of London, UK. He carried out further postgraduate research at the Karolinska Institute, Stockholm, Sweden, where he was awarded his research MD.

Dr Montgomery is one of the foremost researchers in the treatment of depression and anxiety disorders. He has a great breadth of experience in the field of psychotropic medicine with seminal work in depression, anxiety disorders, suicide prevention and schizophrenia. His reputation was established with his early work on improving the methodology of clinical trials. His numerous placebo-controlled studies in the long-term treatment of depression and anxiety have set the standard for investigations in the field. The Montgomery and Asberg Depression Rating Scale is now recognised as the most sensitive instrument for measuring efficacy. He has published more than 400 research reports and reviews and has authored 26 books.

Dr Montgomery has served on the executive committee and councils of numerous national and international scientific societies. He has been President of the British Association of Psychopharmacology and President of the European College of Neuropsychopharmacology. He has considerable experience in the licensing of treatments and has served for many years on the Committee on Safety of Medicines in the UK in the past.

Dr Montgomery is editor of *International Clinical Psychopharmacology* and *European Neuropsychopharmacology* as well as serving on the editorial board of numerous other scientific journals.

Author biography

Dr Stuart A Montgomery [illegible]

Chapter 1

The changing concept of generalised anxiety disorder

Generalised anxiety disorder (GAD) is commonly regarded to be the key anxiety disorder. How it acquired this position can be traced, to some extent, to the changes that have occurred over time in the development of the *Diagnostic and Statistical Manual* (DSM) of the American Psychiatric Association which is the main tool used for diagnosis.[1–5] This system, which continues to be developed by committee, has been through major changes in the course of successive versions.

The vague notion of anxiety neurosis, put forward by Freud in 1884 to make a separation from neurasthenia but without criteria, was adopted uncritically in the early version of DSM[5] and DSM-II.[6] The concept of neurosis was abandoned as unhelpful in DSM-III[2] where operational criteria for individual anxiety disorders were introduced.

There is a well-recognised tension between those who prefer wider categories of disorders and those who prefer to refine the wider category into smaller contributing components, known familiarly as the difference between lumpers and splitters. When the DSM-III was developed the splitters predominated on the committees and it was decided to recognise panic disorder as a separate category. This left a larger category of a more general sort of anxiety, later named generalised anxiety disorder. Some recognition that GAD was the true inheritor of the anxiety label came when buspirone, which had been investigated for efficacy in placebo-controlled studies in anxiety neurosis,[7,8] was approved in the US by the Food and Drug Administration (FDA) for the treatment of GAD on the grounds that this was the closest equivalent diagnosis.

The evolution of GAD in the DSM system was helped by its recognition in 1980 in DSM-III[2] as a separate disorder defined by a relatively large number of anxiety symptoms, both somatic and psychic, which were required to have persisted for a period of at least 30 days. The definition of GAD in DSM-III appears to match quite closely the concept of GAD as measured on the Hamilton Anxiety Scale[9] in which both psychic and somatic symptoms are well represented. The relatively short duration of the disorder required would allow the inclusion of a number of individuals with short-lived anxiety states as well as a larger group with the more chronic condition. In a radical change of position in the DSM-IIIR[1] categorisation, episodes of anxiety having a duration of less than 6 months were excluded and the diagnosis of GAD reserved exclusively for the persistent, chronic form of the disorder. This development helped identify a group associated with a high degree of suffering and fewer short episodes. GAD in this formulation might still have a waxing and waning character but now on a background of clearly demonstrable chronic persistent anxiety. There is, however, a fairly large group of sufferers of GAD who have discrete episodes of anxiety separated by periods of remission and these are neglected in the current definition. These short-lived, more discrete episodes of anxiety are also associated with considerable disability.[10]

In 1994, the DSM system was again revised (DSM-IV)[4] to redefine GAD focusing on the core psychic symptoms of anxiety (Figure 1.1). This stated that

Current DSM-IV diagnostic criteria for generalised anxiety disorder

A Excessive anxiety and worry (apprehensive expectation) occurring more days than not for at least 6 months, about a number of events or activities

B The person finds it difficult to control worry

C The anxiety and worry are associated with three (or more) of the following six symptoms (with at least some symptoms present for more days than not for the past 6 months)
Note: only one item is required in children
(1) restlessness or feeling keyed up or on edge
(2) being easily fatigued
(3) difficulty concentrating or mind going blank
(4) irritability
(5) muscle tension
(6) sleep disturbance (difficulty falling or staying asleep or restless unsatisfying sleep)

D The focus of the anxiety and worry is not confined to features of another axis 1 disorder

E The anxiety, worry or physical symptoms cause clinically significant distress of impairment in social, occupational or other important areas of functioning

F The disturbance is not due to the direct physiological effects of a substance (eg, a drug of abuse, a medication) or a general medical condition (eg, hyperthyroidism), and does not occur exclusively during a mood disorder, a psychotic disorder or a pervasive developmental disorder

Figure 1.1 Current DSM-IV diagnostic criteria for generalised anxiety disorder.
DSM, Diagnostic and Statistical Manual. Adapted from the American Psychiatric Association.[3]

there had to be excessive anxiety or worry about a number of events or activities accompanied by at least half of a list of symptoms encompassing restlessness or mental tension, fatigue, poor concentration, irritability, muscle tension, sleep disturbance, all occurring for most days over a 6-month period. There is an additional requirement that the worry is difficult to control and causes significant distress or impairment in function.

These frequent changes in diagnostic definitions reflect the pleomorphic nature of anxiety and the question arises as to whether the committee have correctly defined GAD. The rapid changes in what is required to fulfil the diagnosis of GAD have left many doctors and their patients behind; many doctors are still in the habit of using a broader number of anxiety symptoms to define the condition. Questions also remain concerning the almost complete exclusion of somatic symptoms to help define GAD since autonomic symptoms and pain are frequent in GAD. The diagnosis of GAD as currently defined in the DSM may not adequately define this serious disorder. There have been some suggestions that major depressive disorder (MDD) and GAD might be merged because of the number of overlapping symptoms. However, the data from follow-up studies carried out in Zurich[10] show that the more serious overlap of symptoms occurs not with MDD but with bipolar depression.

The studies investigating the efficacy of treatments for GAD were all carried out using the DSM criteria. Health statistics are gathered using the *International Classification of Diseases* (ICD). This is potentially confusing as the descriptions in the current ICD version, ICD-10,[11] do not exactly match those of DSM and tend to be more loosely defined. Strictly speaking there is no direct evidence of efficacy of treatment of GAD defined by ICD-10 but the categorisation is sufficiently close to assume that efficacy of treatment established using DSM-IV probably also applies to ICD-10.

Chapter 2

How common is generalised anxiety disorder?

Generalised anxiety disorder (GAD) as currently defined is a very common disorder with an estimated lifetime prevalence reported in European and US epidemiological studies of 4–6% and a 12-month prevalence of 1.5–2% (Figure 2.1). Prevalence estimates inevitably vary depending on the strictness of the diagnostic definition used to define a case. Higher estimates can be expected

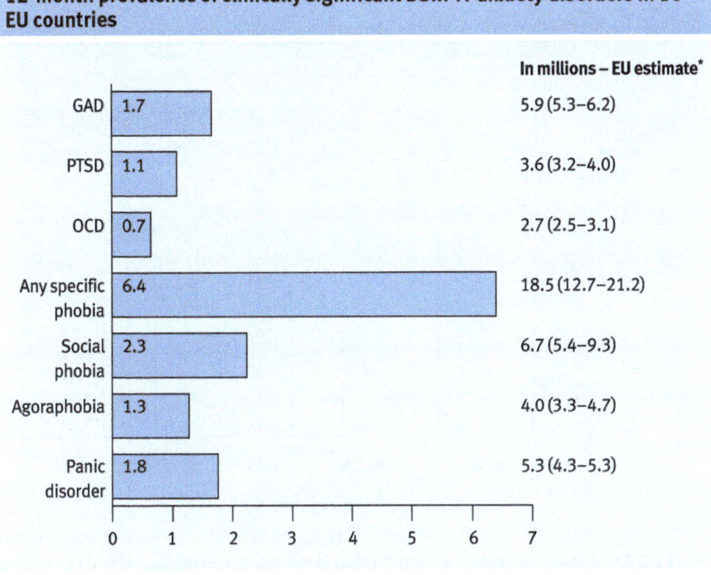

Figure 2.1 12-month prevalence of clinically significant DSM-IV anxiety disorders in 16 EU countries. EU, European Union; GAD, generalised anxiety disorder; OCD, obsessive–compulsive disorder; PTSD, post-traumatic stress disorder. *Total EU population (aged 18–65) = 301.7 million; estimates were based on $n = 156\,000$. Adapted from Wittchen et al.[12]

if the less demanding one-month minimum duration criterion is applied.[2] The later, more restrictive criteria of DSM-IV appear to identify a smaller, more stable, possibly more homogeneous group, albeit one where the presentation is somewhat skewed in the direction of psychic symptomatology. As with other depressive and anxiety disorders, there is an over-representation of women, in whom the disorder is observed twice as frequently as in men.

Prevalence estimates of GAD are particularly high if they are based on a primary care population rather than the general population (Figure 2.2). It has been estimated that there is a lifetime prevalence of 6–8% in primary care compared with 2% in the community samples. Those with GAD appear to recognise their need for care and are frequent attenders in primary care clinics. In this regard they differ from those with depression – both major depressive disorder (MDD) and bipolar depression – who very frequently do not recognise their need for treatment.

GAD differs from depression and other anxiety disorders in having a late age of onset (Figure 2.3). In other anxiety disorders the average age of onset occurs in the late teens or early twenties. In contrast, GAD has a late average onset of around age 35. This is reflected in the increasing prevalence reported with age. The maximum 12-month prevalence, for example, was not reached in men until

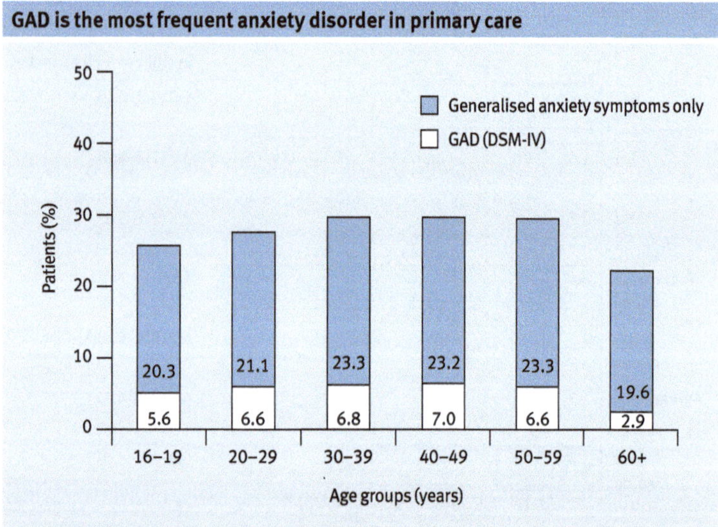

Figure 2.2 GAD is the most frequent anxiety disorder in primary care. DSM, Diagnosic and Statistical Manual; GAD, generalised anxiety disorder. Results from the generalised anxiety disorder in primary care (GAD-P) study showed that a third of patients had some GAD symptoms. Point prevalence among consecutive attenders; $n = 20451$ patients – total assessment. Based on DSM-IV criteria. Adapted from Wittchen et al.[13]

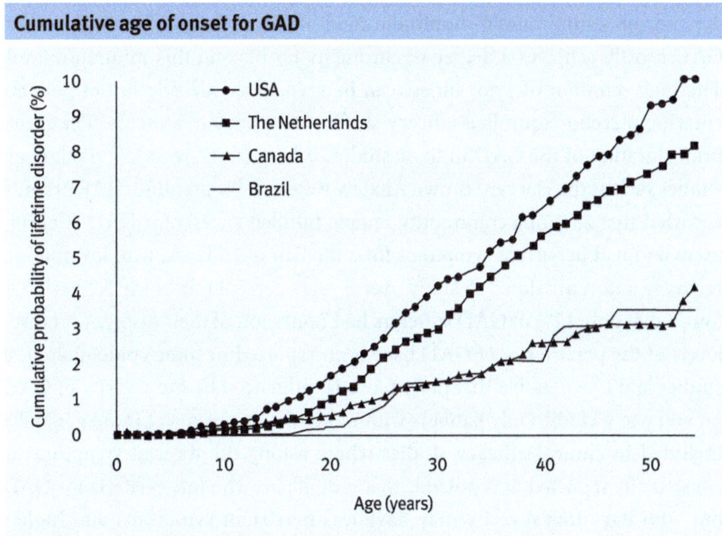

Figure 2.3 Cumulative age of onset for GAD. GAD, generalised anxiety disorder. Age of onset distributions for lifetime generalised anxiety disorder. Data from Kessler et al.[14]

age 65 and in women until age 49.[12] In a small study in a German population the prevalence in those aged over 55 (2.2%) was more than double the prevalence in those under 35 (<1%).[15] This helps explain why GAD is the most frequent psychiatric disorder in those over the age of 55 attending for treatment.[16]

GAD in children and adolescents

Anxiety occurs in both children and adolescents but the diagnosis of GAD is complicated by the difficulty in identifying defined core symptoms. The DSM-IV system acknowledges this problem and has tried to make it easier to fulfil the diagnostic criteria by lowering the number of core supporting symptoms required from three of six to only one of six. Even with these much more flexible criteria the prevalence of GAD in children and adolescents appears to be very low. Because of the variation in the diagnostic requirements it is problematic to regard GAD in children or adolescents as the same disorder as in adults. The course of illness is more variable and less predictable in younger people than in adults where it is mostly a long-term disorder. This suggests that it is not quite the same disorder.

Course of GAD in adults

GAD is defined as a long-term and largely persistent disorder. By definition, it is a disorder the diagnosis of which, in addition to certain symptoms, depends on a minimum 6-month duration of illness that is chronic; however, GAD mostly achieves a degree of chronicity far beyond this minimum level. The long duration of prior illness can be seen in the description of patients entering placebo-controlled efficacy studies of various treatments. The mean prior duration of the GAD in these studies is long (6–17 years).[17,18] Follow-up studies such as the Harvard Brown Anxiety Research Programme (HARP) study reported that 25% of a community sample fulfilled criteria for GAD at enrolment and had persistent symptoms for a median of 16 years, with low rates of recovery and remission.[19] A study over 3 years carried out in the Netherlands found that only 12% of GAD sufferers had remission of their disorder.[20] Lower levels of the persistence of GAD have been reported in some epidemiological studies and it is possible that persistence is influenced by the severity of GAD on entry to a study. Only patients with moderate or severe GAD are generally included in clinical efficacy studies where a long duration of symptoms is consistently reported. It is possible that individuals who meet criteria for GAD but who have low severity may have less persistent symptoms and higher remission rates. This would contribute to the perception that the course of GAD is long term but that it may run an episodic course.

The long-term outcome of GAD depends partly on whether the individual receives appropriate and adequate treatment. The data in this respect are somewhat mixed. The general picture has been one of undertreatment, for example it has been reported that only 40% of those recruited to clinical efficacy studies in GAD had received prior treatment despite the very long prior duration of illness.[17] Similar figures are reported from a recent survey of 136 primary care practices in Norway, which found that the rate of identification of GAD was low and of those who were recognised only 36% were treated.[21]

Even when patients receive treatment, the quality of care provided is uneven. Much of the treatment offered has not been established as effective. As few as 11% of individuals with GAD appear to be offered medication while 22% are provided with information only, 35% counselling and 13% counselling or help with practical issues.[22]

Chapter 3

Presenting features of generalised anxiety disorder

The key symptoms of GAD defined in the current version of the DSM are: excessive anxiety and worry that are difficult to control and present for most days for a period of 6 months or more. However, the primary complaints that bring patients to seek medical attention are frequently at variance with this picture.

Anxiety symptoms, while present, are frequently not the primary complaint in patients with GAD presenting in primary care (Figure 3.1), which is unfortunate as those presenting with anxiety symptoms stand a better chance of their GAD being detected. Since those with GAD complain mostly about somatic symptoms and pain it is unfortunate that these are not included as important diagnostic features.

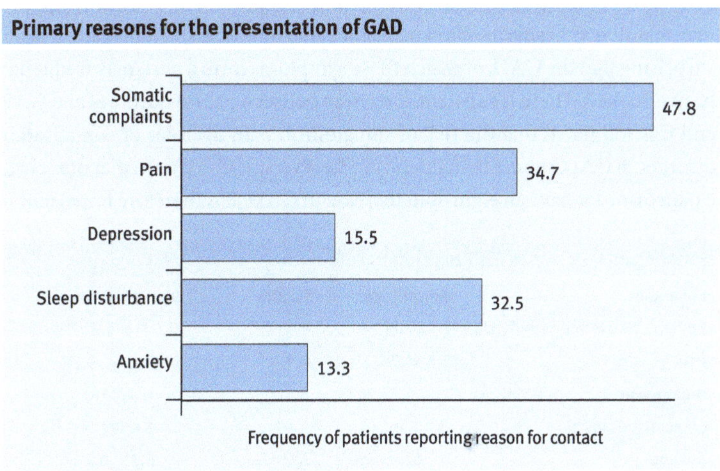

Figure 3.1 Primary reasons for presentation of GAD. GAD, generalised anxiety disorder. Data from Wittchen et al.[13]

Somatic symptoms

It is clear that in primary care the majority of those with GAD present with various somatic complaints (Figure 3.2). In a study carried out in primary care in Germany,[13] anxiety was the primary complaint in only 13.3% of patients with GAD. Approximately 48% presented with various somatic symptoms, and approximately 35% with pain symptoms. These somatic symptoms (Figure 3.3) are often not recognised as being part of GAD and contribute to the poor recognition rate of pure GAD in primary care. This failure to detect GAD leads to a large number of investigations aimed at exploring possible physical conditions while the GAD is overlooked. Approximately half of the direct costs of managing GAD can be attributed to the cost of these investigations.

GAD is associated with an increased risk of a variety of physical disorders. These include irritable bowel syndrome, coronary heart disease, diabetes and arthritis.[23] Careful investigation is needed when these disorders present for treatment in order to identify the possible presence of GAD. For example, in a series of patients investigated for atypical chest pain 23% had GAD.[24] In another study of chest pain half the patients with a normal angiogram were found to have GAD.[25] GAD is conceptualised as an anxiety disorder not as a somatic disorder and a presentation with predominantly physical symptoms is a significant negative predictor of recognition of GAD.

Pain

Pain is a presenting symptom of GAD in 35% of cases. The painful symptoms may manifest as headache, chest pain, gut pain, or muscle and joint pain. It is not surprising that the GAD, of which these symptoms form a part, may frequently be overlooked. There is substantial overlap between pain syndromes and GAD and it is estimated that the risk of somatoform pain disorder or somatisation disorder in GAD is more than doubled. The reverse is also true in that those with a pain disorder have an eight-fold increase in GAD. It is therefore important to

Presenting features of GAD in primary care

Complaint	Percentage	Odds ratio	95% confidence
Somatic illness and complaints	47.8	1.5	1.3–1.8
Pain	34.7	1.3	1.1–1.6
Depression	15.5	8.6	6.8–11.0
Sleep disturbance	32.5	8.4	6.4–11.0
Anxiety	13.3	8.0	6.2–10.2

Figure 3.2 Presenting features of GAD in primary care. GAD, generalised anxiety disorder. Data from Wittchen et al.[13]

Somatic symptoms associated with GAD	
Psychic	**Somatic**
Nervousness, irritability, worrying	Muscle tightness or stiffness
Restlessness, tension, inability to relax	Headache, back pain
Difficulty concentrating, memory problems	Gastrointestinal symptoms
Anxiety	Cardiovascular
	Respiratory
	Insomnia
	Fatigue

Figure 3.3 Somatic symptoms associated with GAD. GAD, generalised anxiety disorder.

bear both aspects of the disorder in mind when considering choice of treatment. Clearly, a treatment that has a good therapeutic effect on both the anxiety and the pain symptoms should be preferred where both disorders coexist. This is not the case with all the medications that have been shown to be effective in GAD, for example, selective serotonin reuptake inhibitors (SSRIs), buspirone and benzodiazepines are not effective in pain disorders.

Sleep disturbance

It is not always fully appreciated that sleep disturbance is a core feature of GAD and is the presenting complaint in over 30% of patients with GAD. Unfortunately most of the treatments licensed for GAD (eg, SSRIs, serotonin noradrenaline reuptake inhibitors [SNRIs], buspirone) do not target sleep disturbance and may even make the sleep worsen initially. Only one treatment licensed for GAD, pregabalin, has a direct, early and beneficial effect on sleep. Benzodiazepines or other hypnotics are also useful for relieving sleep disturbance but, in practice, are most likely to be given in low doses that are unlikely to have any therapeutic effect on the other symptoms of GAD.

Chapter 4

Comorbidity of generalised anxiety disorder with other conditions

Comorbidity is common with GAD and the majority of patients presenting with GAD also have at least one other diagnosis. Analysis of data from Germany found that comorbidity for any depressive or anxiety disorder was 91.3% (Figure 4.1).[15] This high level of comorbidity is similar to the estimate from the prospective naturalistic follow-up study of patients with anxiety disorders from the Harvard Brown Anxiety Disorders Research Program (HARP) where 83% of patients with GAD had another anxiety disorder.[19]

Comorbidity with GAD over 12 months in Germany

Comorbidity	Percentage
Major depressive disorder	59
Somatoform disorder	48.1
Dysthymia	36.2
Specific phobia	29.3
Social anxiety disorder	28.9
Panic disorder	21.5
Nicotine dependence	14
Agoraphobia without panic disorder	11.3
Obssessive–compulsive disorder	10
Alcohol abuse/dependence	6.4
Eating disorder	2.5
Drug abuse/dependence	1.4
Any 1	91.3
Any 2	40.6
Any 3 or more	32.7

Figure 4.1 Comorbidity with GAD over 12 months in Germany. GAD, generalised anxiety disorder. Data taken from Carter et al.[15]

Comorbidity with depression

The most commonly observed comorbidity is with major depressive episodes (both bipolar and unipolar). In the National Comorbidity Study (NCS) those with the lifetime prevalence of GAD comorbid with depression was 62%, and 39% reported having depression in the previous 30 days.[26] A high level of comorbidity with depression (59%) was reported in the German study[15] as discussed earlier and was similar to that reported in the ESEMeD study (European Study of Epidemiology of Mental Disorders) where 70% of those with GAD had comorbid MDD in the preceding year.[27]

Those with depression who also have GAD are more likely to suffer a relapse of their disorder and this also applies if the GAD symptoms are subsyndromal. It should be noted that subsyndromal GAD impairs functioning.[19] Comorbidity of GAD and depression may also impair the response to treatment of the depression. Where GAD is comorbid with depression a poor outcome of the GAD is more likely and there is a lower chance of remission.[28,29] Recent data from the Treatment Resistant Depression Group shows that comorbidity with any anxiety disorder including GAD is a predictor of treatment resistance in depression.[30]

Comorbidity with anxiety disorders

There is considerable comorbidity of GAD with other anxiety disorders: social anxiety disorder, specific phobia and panic disorder are found in 20–30% of individuals with GAD.[15] Panic disorder, social and specific phobias, and post-traumatic stress disorder were the most common comorbid anxiety disorders reported in the NCS.[31] There is, of course, a considerable overlap in symptoms among the anxiety disorders. This makes it difficult to separate the different disorders and, unless close attention is paid to whether the two disorders have a different time course, the estimates of comorbidity may in some cases be exaggerated. However, since GAD has a late age of onset and the other anxiety disorders have an early age of onset, it is easier to separate the long-term clinical course of GAD and that of the comorbid disorder.

When GAD is comorbid with other anxiety disorders impairment increases, as does health-seeking behaviour when compared with GAD or the other anxiety disorders alone.[14] The presence of comorbid panic disorder or other anxiety disorders with GAD worsens the outcome despite the increase in health-seeking behaviour.[19] Poor levels of recognition and the failure to provide the appropriate treatment for GAD are also likely to contribute to a poor outcome.

Somatic disorders

GAD is associated with somatic symptoms and it is no surprise that there is substantial comorbidity of GAD with a variety of physical disorders. People with GAD have an increased risk of coronary heart disease, hypertension and irritable bowel disease. The risk of having any chronic somatic disease comorbid with GAD is doubled when compared with the healthy population.[23,32] Comorbidity of GAD with a physical disorder raises the level of dysfunction but at the same time appears to lower the level of the recognition of GAD. This is not surprising since the focus of attention of the patient with GAD and the presenting complaints are largely somatic.

GAD is frequently comorbid with both pain and pain disorders. The presenting complaint in patients with GAD is frequently pain, and the odds ratio of having a pain syndrome is high. As with other somatic complaints, the focus on pain by the patient tends to divert the doctor away from considering the presence of GAD. The presence of pain or other somatic complaints should lead the clinician to consider the possible presence of GAD in the differential diagnosis rather than neglect this possibility.

Identifying GAD and comorbid conditions

Although primary care doctors recognise a clear impairment due to the presence of a mental disorder they appear to recognise pure GAD less readily than, for example, pure major depressive disorder (MDD).[13] The frequent comorbidity of GAD can complicate the diagnosis and this may partly explain the relatively low recognition rate for GAD in primary care.

Most anxiety disorders have an early age of onset and any comorbid depression tends to develop later. The opposite is true with GAD. The depression tends to develop first and then later comorbid GAD may arise. This is not unlike the development of bipolar disorder where MDD develops first and then some time later the bipolar disorder becomes evident with the development of hypomania or mania. Since there is evidence that there is a close overlap of GAD with bipolar disorder, this raises the question of whether the late development of GAD is related to bipolar disorder.

Anxiety symptoms are common in MDD and many patients with GAD may fulfil diagnostic criteria for MDD so that it is sometimes difficult to separate the two disorders. The time course of each of the disorders (MDD or GAD) can provide guidance; if both disorders have exactly the same time course it is likely that only one disorder (probably depression) is present. If, however, the time courses of the anxiety or depressive symptoms differ and they are not contemporary at all times then it is more likely that two separate disorders of MDD and GAD are present. In these cases there may well be an advantage in prescribing a treatment that is effective in both conditions. Since some selective serotonin reuptake inhibitors (SSRIs) and serotonin noradrenaline reuptake inhibitors (SNRIs) have been found to be effective in both MDD and GAD, these treatments should be used preferentially in the presence of an obvious comorbidity.

The same principle applies in separating GAD from other comorbid disorders (eg, irritable bowel syndrome, respiratory disorders, cardiac disorders, pain disorders). Here, too, separation of the time course of each disorder is helpful. Clearly where an effective therapy for GAD exists that is also effective in treating the comorbid disorder, that treatment will be preferred.

Chapter 5

Burden of generalised anxiety disorder

GAD is associated with major functional impairment in work (Figure 5.1) or social activity and impairs the quality of life. The requirements to meet the diagnosis of GAD according to the DSM-IV take account of this reduction in function: it is necessary to establish that the individual suffers either clinically significant distress or impairment in social, occupational or other areas of functioning. The effects of the disorder are detrimental to individual sufferers but the disorder also affects their families and the cost to society is high. Yet the rates of recognition and treatment are unusually low for a disorder with such far-reaching consequences.

GAD is a long-term disorder that is associated with increased disability and a reduced quality of life. The disability, identified in terms of work impairment and distress, appears to be similar in young adults regardless of the defining duration of the disorder (eg, 2 weeks, 1 month, 3 months, 6 months).[33] Social impairment increased with the longer duration of GAD but the data from the Zurich study[10,33] suggest that the overall burden of illness is similar in short and longer durations of GAD.

Studies to assess disability in GAD carried out in the US, Europe and Australia come to very similar conclusions. In the US, one study found that scores on all domains measured by the Short-Form (SF-36) Health Survey (eg, mental health, social function, role function, general health, bodily pain) were significantly lower in GAD compared with controls without GAD.[34] These impairments in quality of life persisted despite treatment of varying kinds received by some 60% of those followed up in the study. Similar results are reported in other studies in the US, with higher levels of disability recorded in patients with GAD when compared with those without the disorder.[35] Moreover, in the US, some low-income groups with GAD also have higher levels of disability when compared with those with other psychiatric disorders.[36]

The disability associated with major depressive disorder (MDD) is now recognised as being greater than with many other chronic physical disorders. The disability associated with GAD has been recognised more recently. Social and work impairment in GAD was found to be in line with that reported in MDD in both the US[37] and Germany.[38] Where there was comorbidity of GAD with MDD there was even greater disability compared to the pure disorders. However, GAD does occur on its own, independently of MDD.

GAD itself is associated with high levels of disability and impairment in daily functioning. The impairment increases with increased severity of the GAD.[39] The level of impairment of pure GAD is in line with that observed in depression. However, this high level of impairment in GAD is increased further when comorbidity with depression supervenes.[38] This increased impairment in GAD, together with the extra comorbidity with depression, also raised the suicide rate above that observed for either GAD or depression alone. A study in the US reported similar results; in patients with pure GAD the disability and impairment were the same as in patients with pure depressive disorders although the disability in the comorbid group was still higher.[40] As might be expected, the severity of the disorder plays its part and the burden of GAD has been shown to be related to the severity of the psychic and somatic symptoms as measured on the Hamilton Anxiety Scale.

The pattern of symptoms of GAD are similar in elderly patients to those seen in younger patients as was reported in the only placebo-controlled study of GAD in those aged over 65 years.[41] However, the anxiety symptoms seem to be more severe in older patients, compared with younger patients, and the impairment and disability consequently greater.[42]

Suicide risk and the burden of GAD

The burden of GAD should include the dangers inherent in the disorder. GAD is a risk factor for suicide as well as for suicidal thoughts and attempted suicide. In the Harvard Brown Anxiety Research Programme (HARP) study on GAD Keller et al[19] reported that in 7% of the sample who entered the study suicide attempts had occurred. The suicide attempt rate was higher (15%) when GAD was comorbid with depression, but both disorders are independent risk factors. The rate of completed suicide in depression is high, estimated to be a lifetime risk of at least 15%. This rate is reported to be even higher in those with increased anxiety symptoms or in those with comorbid GAD or panic disorder. For example, in primary care around 25% of patients with pure GAD and 64% of those with comorbid GAD and MDD had suicidality (thoughts, plans or actual suicide attempts) in the preceding month.[13]

Costs of GAD

Most of the estimates of the cost burden of anxiety disorders have not separated GAD from the other anxiety disorders. However in those studies that focused on GAD the costs are reported to be high. In a primary care sample in the US, for example, the median medical care costs per year for patients with GAD were $US 2375 compared with $US 1448 in those without GAD. The combination of pain and GAD appears to be particularly costly and the medical care costs were highest for those who had GAD in combination with pain that caused interference in function.[43] Similar increases in the direct costs of GAD have been reported in France where the costs were higher in the presence of any comorbidity.[44] These costs were due to clinic visits, hospitalisations, accident and emergency costs, internal medicine consultations, and diagnostic and laboratory tests. The costs of medication represented only 5% of the total costs.

Attendance rates in primary care are three to four times higher than expected from the prevalence data and this frequent attendance contributes to the costs of the disorder. An increase in emergency department visits compared with other axis I disorders is also reported.[45] The high direct cost of managing GAD, particularly when levels of pain are high, relates in large part to the costs of investigating the physical symptoms with which patients present.

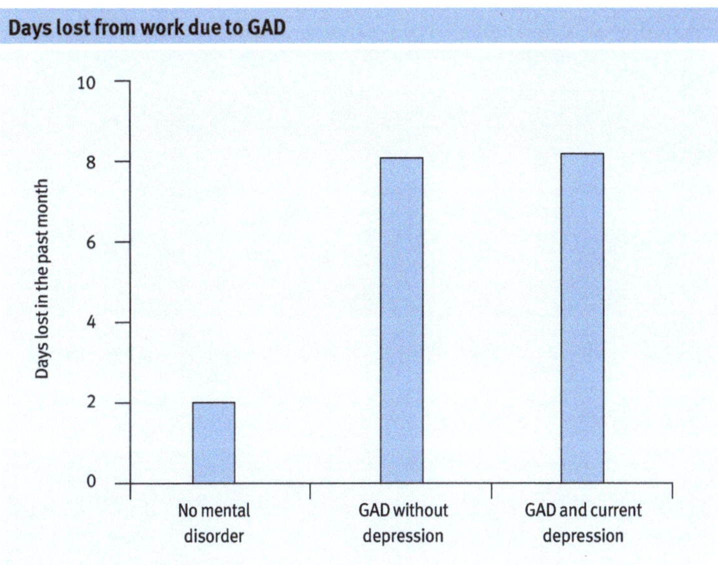

Figure 5.1 Days lost from work due to GAD. GAD, generalised anxiety disorders. Reproduced with permission from Wittchen et al.[46]

The failure to recognise and properly treat GAD has the effect of greatly increasing the number of investigations, many of them potentially unnecessary. One study over a 12-month period found that, although over half the sample with GAD had received some form of intervention including psychotherapy, social support and counselling, evidence-based medical interventions (ie, medicine or cognitive–behavioural therapy) were used in only 6.9% of the sample.[22] The failure to provide appropriate treatment prolongs the disorder, the accompanying pain and somatic suffering and repeat clinic visits, and therefore further increases the direct costs.

The indirect costs of GAD include the loss of work days and also inefficient work days (Figure 5.1). A 50% reduction of work productivity and an increase in days not working are reported.[38] Further costs are incurred in providing the necessary appropriate financial and social support for sufferers and their dependants. Nor should the cost burden of early retirement be overlooked. Both direct and indirect costs of GAD are high which emphasises the need for better recognition and effective treatment.

Chapter 6

Measuring the severity of generalised anxiety disorder

The most widely used instrument for measuring the severity of GAD is the Hamilton Anxiety (HAM-A) scale (Figure 6.1).[9]

The HAM-A comprises a mixture of psychic anxiety symptoms, somatic anxiety symptoms and depressive symptoms. The major subscales used are the psychic anxiety and the somatic anxiety subscales to measure possible differential effects of treatments. The psychic anxiety symptoms on the scale, which measure worries, irritability, fears, fatigability, poor concentration, as well as the somatic symptom of insomnia, are currently used to define GAD; the somatic symptoms which include pain, cardiovascular, respiratory, gastrointestinal, genitourinary, autonomic and other somatic symptoms have been somewhat overlooked. This neglect stems to some extent from the rush to use selective serotonin reuptake inhibitors (SSRIs) and serotonin noradrenaline reuptake inhibitors (SNRIs) that have been shown to be effective in GAD but which may not work well on these somatic symptoms. A reappraisal of this strategy is long overdue.

Other assessment scales that have been used both in GAD and in other anxiety disorders include the anxiety subscale of the Hospital Anxiety and Depression Scale[47] which has proved the most useful in identifying effective treatments compared with placebo. For example, this self-rating scale proved capable of demonstrating the efficacy of venlafaxine in all five placebo-controlled studies in GAD, whereas the HAM-A showed its efficacy in only three of the five studies. This was possibly because venlafaxine had a differential benefit on the psychic symptoms of anxiety rather than on the somatic ones. The Covi Anxiety (Figure 6.2) and Raskin Depression scales are sometimes applied particularly at the beginning of a treatment study in order to establish whether anxiety or depressive symptoms are the more predominant.[48,49] Efficacy on the three-item Covi scale has been reported but it appears less sensitive than other scales.

Hamilton Anxiety rating scale

All items scored 0–4

0 = none, 1 = mild, 2 = moderate, 3 = severe, 4 = very severe

1 Anxious mood
Worries, anticipation of the worst, apprehension (fearful anticipation), irritability

2 Tension
Feelings of tension, fatigability, inability to relax, startle response, moved to tears easily, trembling, feelings of restlessness

3 Fears
Dark, strangers, being left alone, large animals, traffic, crowds

4 Insomnia
Difficulty in falling asleep, broken sleep and fatigue on waking, dreams, nightmares, night terrors

5 Intellectual (cognitive)
Difficulty in concentration, poor memory

6 Depressed mood
Loss of interest, lack of pleasure in hobbies, depression, early waking, diurnal swing

7 General somatic (muscular)
Muscular pains, aches, stiffness, twitching, clonic jerks, grinding of teeth, unsteady voice

8 General somatic (sensory)
Tinnitus, blurring of vision, hot and cold flushes, feelings of weakness, pricking sensations

9 Cardiovascular symptoms
Tachycardia, palpitations, pain in chest, throbbing of vessels, fainting feelings, missing beat

10 Respiratory symptoms
Pressure or constriction in chest, choking feelings, sighing, dyspnoea

11 Gastrointestinal symptoms
Difficulty in swallowing, wind, dyspepsia, pain before and after meal, burning sensations, fullness, water brash, nausea, vomiting, sinking feelings, 'working' in abdomen, borborygmi, looseness of bowels, loss of weight, constipation

12 Genitourinary symptoms
Frequency and/or urgency of micturition: amenorrhoea, menorrhagia, development of frigidity, premature ejaculation, loss of libido, impotence

13 Autonomic symptoms
Dry mouth, flushing, pallor, tendency to sweat, giddiness, tension, headache, raising of hair

14 Behaviour at interview (general)
Tense, not relaxed, fidgiting hands, picking fingers, clenching, tics, restlessness, pacing, tremor of hands, furrowed brow, strained face, increased muscular tone, sighing respirations, facial pallor

Figure 6.1 Hamilton Anxiety rating scale. Adapted from Hamilton.[9]

Covi-Anxiety Scale

All items scored 1–5
1 = not at all, 2 = somewhat, 3 = moderately, 4 = considerably, 5 = very much

1 Verbal report
Feels nervous shaky, jittery, jumpy, suddenly, scared for no reason, fearful, apprehensive, tense or keyed up, has to avoid certain things, places, activities because of getting frightened, finds it hard to keep mind on a task

2 Behaviour
Appears frightened, shaking, restless apprehensive, jumpy, jittery

3 Somatic complaints
Unjustified sweating, trembling, heart pounding or racing, trouble getting breath, hot or cold spells, restless sleep, going unjustifiably more frequently to bathroom, discomfort at pit of stomach, lump in throat

Figure 6.2 Covi-Anxiety Scale. Adapted from Lipman et al.[48]

In addition to the scales measuring specific aspects and symptoms of GAD it is customary to make a global assessment of severity of the disorder. The Clinician's Global Scale for Severity (CGI-S) and the Clinician's Global Impressions Scale for Change (CGI-C) (Figure 6.3)[50] are used routinely and successfully in studies investigating efficacy. Several measures of impairment or disability have also been developed, of which the most sensitive and the most widely used is the Sheehan Disability Scale (SDS) (Figure 6.4), recently reviewed.[51]

Clinical Global Impression Scale

1 Severity
1 = normal, not at all ill, 2 = borderline ill, 3 = mildly ill, 4 = moderately ill, 5 = markedly ill, 6 = severely ill, 7 = among the most extremely ill patients

2 Improvement/Change
1 = very much improved, 2 = much improved, 3 = minimally improved, 4 = no change, 5 = minimally worse, 6 = much worse, 7 = very much worse

Figure 6.3 Clinical Global Impression Scale. Adapted from Guy.[50]

Sheehan Disability Scale

A brief, patient-rated measurement of disability and impairment.
Please mark ONE circle for each scale

Work*/School
The symptoms have disrupted your work/school work

Not at all	Mildly			Moderately			Markedly			Extremely
0	1	2	3	4	5	6	7	8	9	10

☐ I have not worked/studied at all during the past week for reasons unrelated to the disorder.

*Work includes paid, unpaid volunteer work or training

Social life
The symptoms have disrupted your social life/leisure activities

Not at all	Mildly			Moderately			Markedly			Extremely
0	1	2	3	4	5	6	7	8	9	10

Family life/Home responsibilities
The symptoms have disrupted your family life/home responsibilities

Not at all	Mildly			Moderately			Markedly			Extremely
0	1	2	3	4	5	6	7	8	9	10

Days lost

☐ On how many days in the last week did your symptoms cause you to miss school or work or leave you unable to carry out your normal daily responsibilities?

Days unproductive

☐ On how many days in the last week did you feel so impaired by your symptoms that, even though you went to school or work, your productivity was reduced?

Figure 6.4 Sheehan Disability Scale.

Chapter 7

Pharmacological treatments

The changes over time in the criteria used to diagnose GAD make it difficult to generalise the findings on efficacy from early studies where the selected patient samples fulfilled earlier criteria focusing on short prior duration of the condition. These studies would include an undetermined but substantial proportion of patients in whom the GAD was of short duration. Relating the results to GAD as currently defined by a prolonged prior duration is complicated. Caution is therefore needed in assessing the efficacy of some of the earlier treatments where studies were carried out in patient samples with short duration GAD.

Serotonin reuptake inhibitors

The selective serotonin reuptake inhibitors (SSRIs) are thought to exert their therapeutic effect via their action in blocking the reuptake of serotonin (5-hydroxytryptamine or 5-HT) at the synapse. While this applies broadly to all the SSRIs there are considerable pharmacological differences between members of this group of drugs. Most have minor effects on other transmitters such as noradrenaline or dopamine, as well as serotonin, with the most selective being citalopram and escitalopram. Some of these different actions may influence the choice of medication as preferred treatment for particular conditions. For example, fluoxetine in addition to its serotonin reuptake inhibition activity acts as an agonist of 5-HT_{2C}. It is this activity that may be the source of the increase in anxiety early in treatment that is often seen with fluoxetine. This may account for the failure of fluoxetine to separate from placebo in many of the studies of GAD. Fluoxetine inhibits cytochrome P450 (CYP) isoenzymes 2D6 and 3A4 which alter the metabolism of some medications used concomitantly. The active metabolite of fluoxetine, norfluoxetine, has a long elimination half-life so that the drug persists for some 3–5 weeks after termination of treatment. Paroxetine has some anticholinergic properties which may produce a sedative effect and can impair cognitive function. It inhibits CYP2D6 isoenzymes which can increase the plasma levels of some treatments used concomitantly. Sertraline has some activity in inhibiting reuptake of dopamine, an action that has been suggested could increase anxiety at the start of treatment and it also binds to sigma receptors. Its effects on adrenoceptors may lead to mydriasis and dry mouth. It shares the disadvantage of some of the other SSRIs in producing inhibition of CYP2D6. Citalopram, which has not been properly investigated in GAD, is a selective inhibitor of the reuptake of serotonin which lacks important effects on noradrenaline, dopamine or muscarinic receptors, giving it a relatively low side-effect burden. Like other SSRIs, escitalopram, which is the active *S*-enantiomer of citalopram, binds to the serotonin transporter to produce serotonin reuptake inhibition but in addition to binding to the primary site it also binds to the allosteric binding site of the serotonin transporter. It is thought that this additional augmenting effect is behind the superior efficacy reported with escitalopram as an antidepressant.[52,53]

The SSRIs are effective antidepressants and some, but not all, have been shown to be effective in treating anxiety disorders such as panic disorder or social anxiety disorder. For the treatment of GAD, however, only escitalopram, paroxetine and sertraline have been shown to be effective at a level recognised by licensing authorities. All three medications are established antidepressants and since depressive symptoms are frequently a part of GAD the possibility of their exerting a therapeutic effect via an antidepressant action has to be addressed. To demonstrate a direct effect on the GAD independent of the efficacy in depression, patients with comorbid major depression have had to be excluded from the efficacy studies.

Paroxetine

Paroxetine was the first SSRI to be investigated and licensed for the treatment of GAD. The studies supporting the regulatory submission were comparisons with placebo but paroxetine has since been included as an active comparator in subsequent studies of other potential treatments for GAD so that some estimate of its relative place in treatment is possible.

Two studies in short-term treatment of GAD patients without significant comorbidity, one having a flexible dose (20–50 mg)[54] and the other comparing fixed doses of 20 mg and 40 mg with placebo,[55] showed that paroxetine was effective in treating GAD. In the flexible dose study the efficacy appeared late at 6 weeks. The rate of response on placebo in the study was high (56%) compared with paroxetine (72%). There is a risk in flexible dose studies that the dose rises carry an extra placebo effect which may contribute to the high placebo response that is frequently observed in this type of study. In the fixed dose study both paroxetine 20 mg and paroxetine 40 mg were associated with higher levels of responders (62% and 68%) than placebo (46%) measured on the Hamilton Anxiety A (HAM-A) rating scale. The response was mainly seen on the psychic symptoms of anxiety and paroxetine did not seem to be effective on the somatic symptom subscale of the HAM-A. The efficacy of paroxetine was also seen in the advantage compared with placebo on the measures of disability applied in this study. The efficacy demonstrated in these two positive, short-term, placebo-controlled studies was further strengthened by the positive result from with paroxetine in preventing relapse over 24 weeks, shown in the long-term relapse-prevention study (Figure 7.1).[56]

Some indication of the relative place of paroxetine compared with other SSRIs is provided by later studies where it was included as a reference medication. For example, it was included as a reference in a study of escitalopram, which investigated doses of 5 mg, 10 mg and 20 mg compared with placebo (Figure 7.2).[17] Both doses of escitalopram that were shown to be effective were reported as superior to paroxetine though the evidence, coming from different analyses, is not strong. The failure of paroxetine to separate from placebo in this study suggests that the study may have been underpowered but nevertheless provides some indication that paroxetine may not be the most effective treatment for GAD.

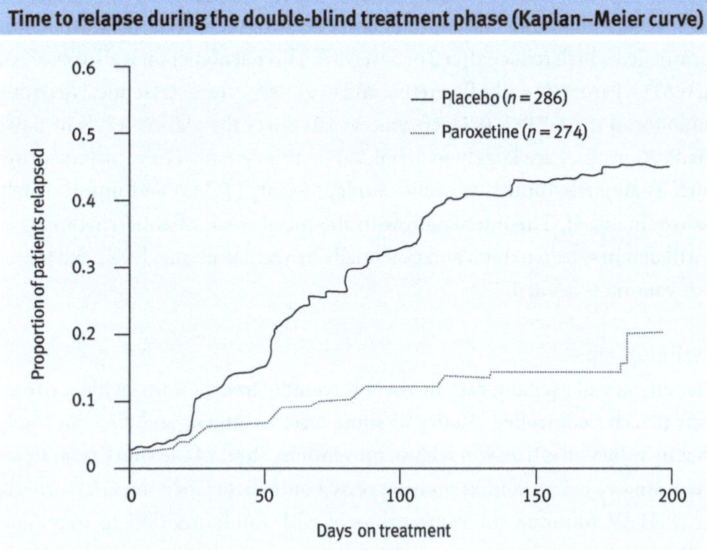

Figure 7.1 Time to relapse during the double-blind phase (Kaplan–Meier curve). Reproduced with permission from Stocchi et al.[56]

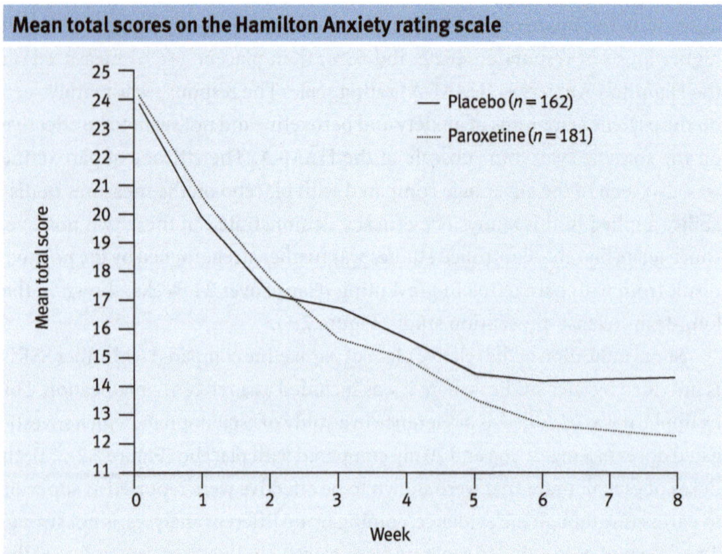

Figure 7.2 Mean total scores on the Hamilton Anxiety rating scale. Adapted from Pollack et al.[54]

Paroxetine has other disadvantages. In the treatment of depression it is associated with marked discontinuation effects in the week after treatment is terminated which reduce after 2 or 3 weeks.[57] This phenomenon is also observed in GAD.[58] Paroxetine, like fluoxetine and to a lesser extent sertraline, is a strong inhibitor of the CYP 2D6 isoenzyme which raises the plasma levels of those medications that are largely metabolised by this system. These include drugs such as antiarrhythmics, tricyclic antidepressants (TCAs) and unfortunately paroxetine itself. The interaction with the metabolism of antiarrhythmics in particular may lead to high and potentially dangerous plasma levels and therefore caution is needed.

Escitalopram

The efficacy of escitalopram in GAD is soundly based on the evidence from four placebo-controlled studies of short-term treatment and also one study that investigated efficacy in relapse prevention. Three of the short-term treatment studies carried out in non-depressed outpatients meeting GAD criteria of DSM-IV followed the same protocol with randomisation to treatment with escitalopram 10 mg or placebo following a single-blind placebo run-in period. After 4 weeks the dose of escitalopram or placebo could be raised to 20 mg/day day for a further 4 weeks. The efficacy of escitalopram compared with placebo at endpoint was shown in all three studies on the HAM-A, the primary efficacy scale. Significant efficacy was also shown on the psychic anxiety symptoms subscale of the HAM-A and the Clinical Global Impression (CGI) severity rating which are secondary scales. There was some evidence of an early effect with escitalopram in the first of the three studies[59] but not in the other two (Figure 7.3).

The use of the same protocol in the three studies made it possible to carry out a pooled analysis of the data that supported the efficacy of escitalopram shown in the individual studies, registered on the primary HAM-A scale and all the secondary scales at endpoint.[60] Analysis of subgroups of the patient population established the efficacy of escitalopram in both the moderate and the severe GAD groups, in men and women, and in the older patients aged between 60 and 65. The analysis showed significantly higher remission rates, defined as HAM-A ≤9 or ≤7 on escitalopram than placebo.

Escitalopram was shown in a fixed-dose, placebo- and paroxetine-controlled study to be effective when given in doses of 10 mg or 20 mg but the 5 mg dose did not separate from placebo. It is unusual to detect a difference between

Mean change from baseline in HAM-A total scores by visit (intention to treat, observed cases) and at last observation carried forward

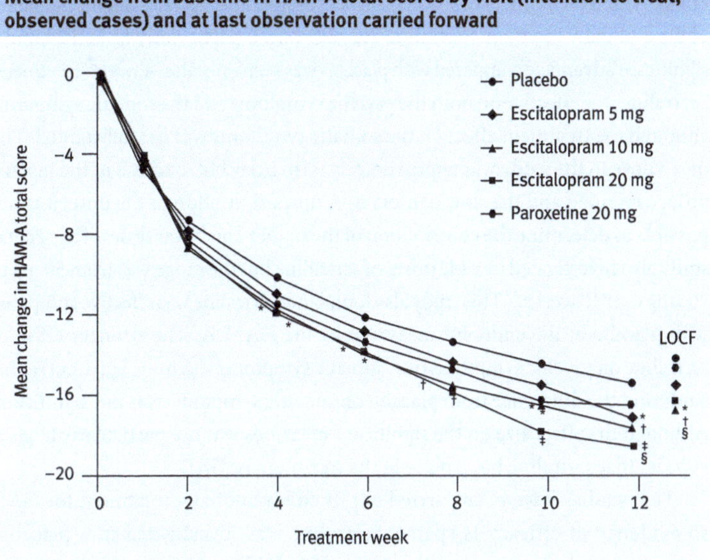

Figure 7.3 Mean change from baseline in HAM-A total scores by visit (intention to treat, observed cases) and at last observation carried forward. HAM-A, Hamilton Anxiety rating scale; LOCF, last observation carried forward. Difference vs placebo, *P<0.05; †P<0.01; ‡P<0.001; difference vs Paroxetine §P<0.05 (analysis of covariance). Reproduced with permission from Baldwin et al.[17]

active medications in a single study and it is therefore interesting that at 12 weeks in the last observation carried forward analysis, which takes account of discontinuations from treatment, escitalopram 10 mg was more effective than paroxetine 20 mg and in the observed case analysis escitalopram 20 mg was better than paroxetine.[17] The efficacy of escitalopram in short-term treatment is supported by efficacy shown in a study of relapse prevention.[61]

Escitalopram appears to be a well-tolerated treatment in GAD in both the short and the long term. There was a low level of unwanted side effects and few patients discontinued treatment for this reason. In the short-term studies nausea, insomnia, fatigue and sexual side effects had an incidence greater than 5% and were twice as frequent as placebo.

Sertraline

The efficacy of sertraline in the treatment of GAD has been shown in two large placebo-controlled studies. In the first of these studies[18] flexible doses from 50 mg to 150 mg of sertraline were compared over 12 weeks with placebo in patients with GAD who did not have current MDD and had only low scores of depressive symptoms. Efficacy was seen at the 12-week endpoint on the primary scale, the HAM-A, and on a variety of secondary measures including assessments of quality of life and daily function. Sertraline did not show a particularly fast effect and a significant advantage compared with placebo was seen only after 4 weeks' treatment. Sertraline was effective on both the psychic symptoms and the somatic symptoms although the treatment effect on the somatic symptoms was less substantial. The mean dose in the study was approximately 95 mg/day but, because of the flexible dosage regimen and the slow conservative upward titration of the dose, it is not possible to determine the contribution of the higher and lower doses. The second study also investigated flexible doses of sertraline but the range was from 50 mg to 200 mg over 10 weeks.[62] This study also found that sertraline was effective compared with placebo at the endpoint measured by the HAM-A. The stronger effect of sertraline on psychic symptoms over somatic symptoms was more apparent in this study and the difference from placebo on somatic symptoms was not significant. Although the effect size on the significant measures was not particularly large, it appears that sertraline has a place in the treatment of GAD.

Few studies have been carried out in children of any treatment for GAD so evidence of efficacy is sparse. Sertraline was investigated in a placebo-controlled study in a very small sample of 22 children with GAD over 9 weeks and appeared to be effective.[63]

Sertraline was well tolerated in the studies in GAD, with side effects similar to those expected for SSRIs.

Serotonin noradrenaline reuptake inhibitors

The serotonin noradrenaline reuptake inhibitors (SNRIs) inhibit the reuptake of both serotonin and noradrenaline though the potency of their action on noradrenaline reuptake varies between members of this group and may depend on dose.

Venlafaxine

The description of venlafaxine as an SNRI is complicated by the dose issue. Only the higher doses of venlafaxine are thought to have a significant effect on noradrenaline reuptake inhibition. Venlafaxine in a dose of 75 mg/day is thought to have only negligible effects on noradrenaline reuptake and to work almost exclusively as an SSRI.

Venlafaxine was introduced in an immediate-release formulation and later an extended-release (ER) formulation. In GAD venlafaxine ER has been found to be effective in a series of short-term and long-term studies in doses of 75, 150 and 225 mg/day compared with placebo (Figure 7.4).[64–67] All three doses of venlafaxine were significantly better than placebo on some or all the measures used in the studies. There appears to be a greater effect on the psychic symptoms of GAD than on the somatic symptoms. The therapeutic benefit of venlafaxine is also seen in its effect in improving social function.[39] The studies

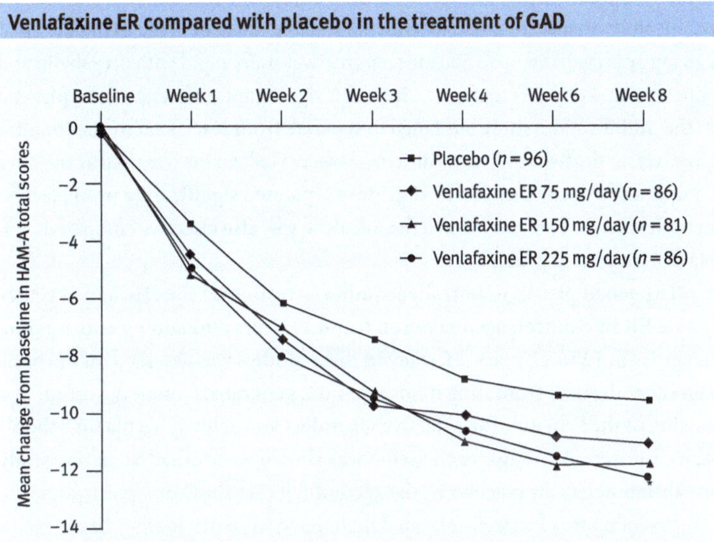

Figure 7.4 Venlafaxine ER compared with placebo in the treatment of GAD. ER, extended release; GAD, generalised anxiety disorder; HAM-A, Hamilton Anxiety rating scale. *$P<0.05$. Reproduced with permission from Rickels et al.[64]

on venlafaxine included several different primary measures of efficacy and a statistical adjustment usually applied to multiple comparisons appears to be lacking. Combined with doubts about possible selective reporting this complicates the interpretation of the results.

The studies did not suggest a significant dose–response relationship and there was an increase in adverse events with higher doses, so that the optimum and target dose should be 75 mg. It seems that in GAD the contribution of noradrenaline reuptake to efficacy is minimal in the short term. The picture is less clear in long-term treatment. A post-hoc meta-analysis[68] of the data from the two 6-month studies[66,67] showed there was a significantly better outcome with increasing doses of venlafaxine. In the short term the adverse events that accompany high doses appear to compromise efficacy but over the long term, when individuals are to some extent habituated to treatment, there may be an advantage in raising the dose.

As with other antidepressants, venlafaxine is not associated with a fast separation from placebo. Of the five placebo-controlled studies submitted to obtain a licence, efficacy on the HAM-A does not suggest a fast response. In a recent study, in which venlafaxine was included as a reference medication, a significant effect for venlafaxine compared with placebo was seen at 2 weeks compared with efficacy seen at 1 week with pregabalin.[69] Similarly in a more recent study that compared placebo and flexible doses of venlafaxine ER up to 225 mg or pregabalin up to 600 mg response was more rapid with pregabalin and appeared at 4 days. Venlafaxine showed a significant difference from placebo in the middle of the study but failed to separate from placebo at the endpoint.[70] However, in the two studies of duloxetine where venlafaxine was used as an active comparator venlafaxine in a flexible dose separated significantly from placebo in both studies. Venlafaxine in a flexible dose was also effective compared with placebo in primary care.[71]

Two small placebo-controlled studies investigated the efficacy of venlafaxine ER in children aged between 6 and 11 years and adolescents ranging in age from 12 to 17 years. Efficacy in these studies was assessed on the basis of a score derived from nine items from the generalised anxiety section of a version of the Schedule for Affective Disorders and Schizophrenia for School-Age Children. Although venlafaxine was shown to be effective in one study the difference from placebo in the second fell just short of significance.[72]

Venlafaxine is less well-tolerated than the SSRIs particularly when given in higher doses. Venlafaxine raises blood pressure and it is recommended that all patients (including adolescents) should be monitored. Venlafaxine also raises total cholesterol at a modest level.

Duloxetine

Duloxetine is the most recent SNRI to be licensed for the treatment of GAD both in the US and in the EU. Its efficacy was established on the basis of three placebo-controlled studies of 9 or 10 weeks' duration. In one study, which investigated duloxetine in fixed doses of 60 mg or 120 mg, both doses showed a significant separation from placebo at 2 weeks.[73] There was no evidence of one dose having a therapeutic advantage over the other, which suggests that the lower dose should be preferred. This could also be interpreted as showing that any additional noradrenaline reuptake inhibition associated with higher doses did not make an obvious contribution to efficacy. The higher doses were less well tolerated with more frequent reports of dizziness, dry mouth and hyperhidrosis, which might be taken as indirect evidence of greater noradrenaline reuptake inhibition activity at higher doses.

Duloxetine was investigated in a flexible dose of 60–120 mg/day in a second study which showed a significantly greater improvement compared with placebo measured on the HAM-A, a higher response rate and greater global improvement.[74] The significantly better response in the duloxetine-treated patients was also seen in the improvement in the functional measures included in the study. There appeared to be no difference in efficacy between venlafaxine, included as a comparator in a further study, and duloxetine, both being significantly better than placebo. Duloxetine was given in a flexible dose of 60–120 mg/day (mean approximately 108 mg/day) and venlafaxine, in a flexible dose of 75–225 mg/day (mean approximately 184 mg/day).[75] Evidence of early response with duloxetine is not convincing. Early separation from placebo at 1 week was seen in only one study.[75] The most frequent adverse events with duloxetine included nausea, decreased appetite, constipation and decreased libido.

Duloxetine is poorly tolerated by some patients even at the lower dose of 60 mg/day and as many as 20% of patients may need their dosage lowered in the first week. The mixed effects repeated measures (MMRM) analysis applied in the studies tends to underestimate the influence of early discontinuations from treatment by assuming that these patients would have continued to improve with the rest of the patients who did not discontinue treatment. Many doctors have adopted the procedure where treatment is started on a low, subtherapeutic dose of duloxetine 30 mg, the dose being later raised to the therapeutic dose of 60 mg (Figure 7.5). This may reduce early dropouts but would also be expected to prolong the time before a significant difference from placebo is observed.

Calcium channel GABA receptor modulators

Pregabalin

Pregabalin modulates the calcium channel in the α_2 subunit of the GABA (γ-aminobutyrate) receptor complex which has the effect of dampening the neurotransmission in excited neurons. The benefits of this action can be seen in the reduction of pain in peripheral and central neuropathy treated with pregabalin in monotherapy, and also in the reduction of partial seizures with pregabalin given as adjunctive treatment.[76,77] Pregabalin has been extensively investigated in eight placebo-controlled studies in GAD and significant efficacy was reported in all but one of these. Pregabalin has currently the largest evidence base of efficacy in the treatment GAD (Figures 7.6–7.9).

Three early 4-week studies investigated the efficacy of pregabalin compared with placebo and with lorazepam in a dose of 6 mg acting as a reference drug. In two of these studies pregabalin in a dose of 600 mg separated significantly from placebo in contrast to lorazepam where only one study showed efficacy. The lower dose of 150mg of pregabalin failed to separate from placebo at the

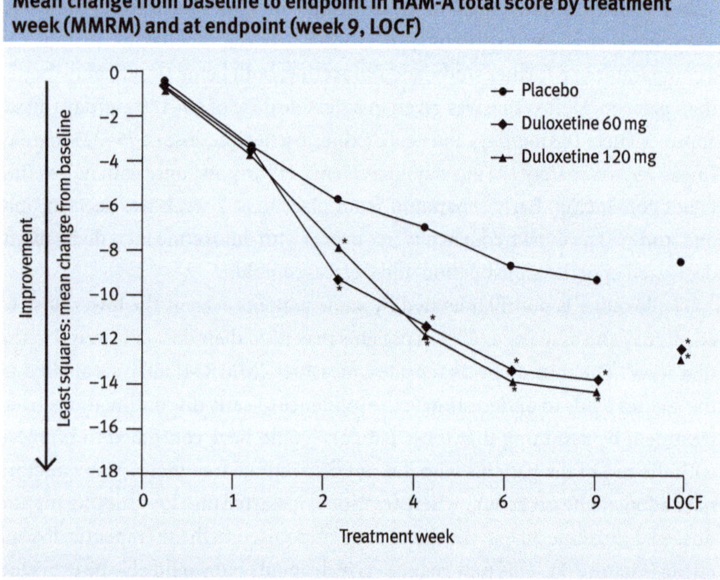

Figure 7.5 Mean change from baseline to endpoint in HAM-A total score by treatment week (MMRM) and at endpoint (week 9, LOCF). *$P \leq 0.001$. HAM-A, Hamilton Anxiety rating scale; LOCF, last observation carried forward; MMRM, mixed effects repeated measures. Reproduced with permission from Koponen et al.[73]

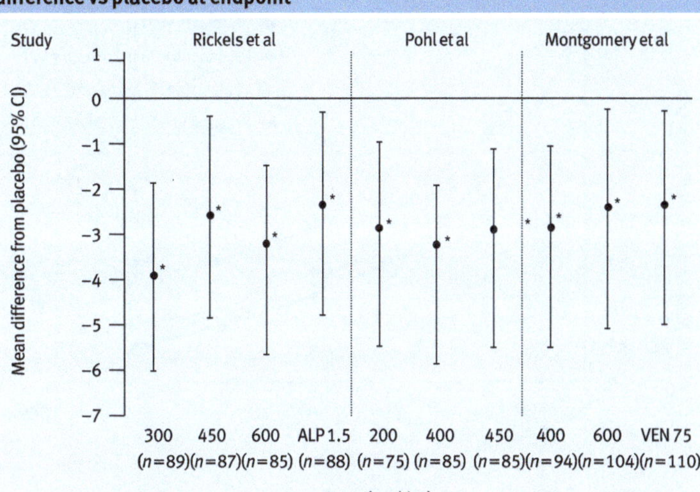

Figure 7.6 Pregabalin efficacy across phase 3 GAD studies: mean (95% CI) HAM-A score difference vs placebo at endpoint. ALP, alprazolam; CI, confidence interval; GAD, generalised anxiety disorder; HAM-A, Hamilton Anxiety rating scale; VEN, venlafaxine. *$P<0.05$ vs placebo. Data taken from Rickels et al.[78] Pohl et al.[79] Montgomery et al.[69]

4-week endpoint in any of these three studies. A pooled analysis of the two positive studies found that pregabalin 150 mg was associated with a significant treatment effect but the effect was obviously less than that of the 600 mg dose.[80,81] Pregabalin 150 mg is therefore considered the subtherapeutic dose. Pregabalin has been found to be effective compared with placebo in a series of studies at daily doses between 200 mg and 600 mg with little difference in efficacy between them so that the target dose of pregabalin for treatment of GAD is usually 300 mg.

A three times daily dosage regimen was used in the early studies but in a later placebo-controlled comparison study a twice daily regimen of pregabalin was as effective.[79] The simpler twice-daily dosage regimen, which is preferred by patients, is therefore recommended.

Two of the later studies included a comparator drug as well as placebo. Alprazolam in a daily dose of 1.5 mg was the reference comparator in one 4-week study investigating three doses of pregabalin (300, 450, and 600 mg/day).[78] All three doses of pregabalin separated early from placebo at 1 week through to the endpoint on the HAM-A scale. The significant treatment effect (difference

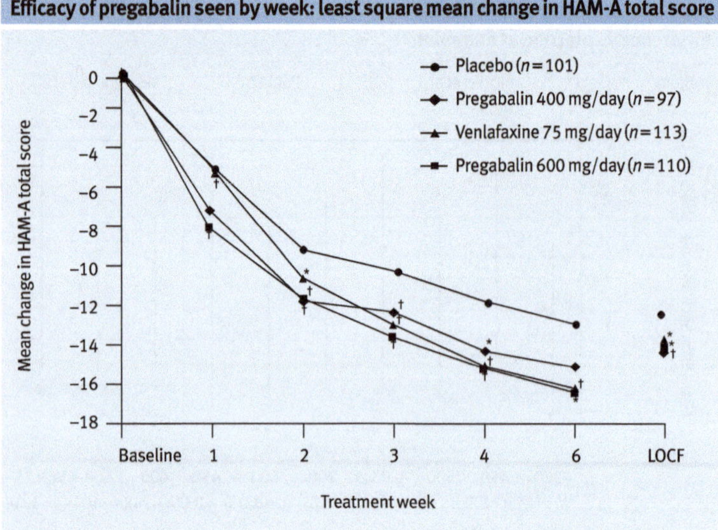

Figure 7.7 Efficacy of pregabalin seen by week 1: least square mean change in HAM-A total score. HAM-A, Hamilton Anxiety rating scale; LOCF, last observation carried forward. *$P<0.05$; †$P<0.01$. Adapted from Montgomery et al.[69]

between active medication and placebo) early in the study with pregabalin at 1 week was nearly twice that seen with alprazolam, which helps to confirm that pregabalin has a fast action in GAD. Efficacy was observed on both the psychic and somatic subscales.

A further placebo-controlled study examined the efficacy of pregabalin in fixed doses of 400 and 600 mg/day with venlafaxine 75 mg/day included as an active comparator. All the treatments separated significantly from placebo at treatment endpoint but the efficacy of pregabalin was seen already after 1 week's treatment whereas venlafaxine had a slower response.[69] The advantage for pregabalin is unlikely to be attributable to the dose of venlafaxine being too low since there is no clear dose–response relationship for venlafaxine.

Further information on the dose issue comes from a placebo-controlled study investigating escalating doses of pregabalin up to 600mg/day and increasing doses of venlafaxine up to 225mg in the XR formulation. Pregabalin showed very early significant separation from both placebo and venlafaxine at 4 days. The efficacy of pregabalin was maintained until the treatment endpoint. The high dose of venlafaxine failed to separate from placebo at treatment endpoint although efficacy was observed midway through the study. This study confirms the very early response seen with pregabalin in the treatment of GAD.[70]

Pregabalin reduces both psychic and somatic symptoms of GAD: pooled analysis from six GAD studies

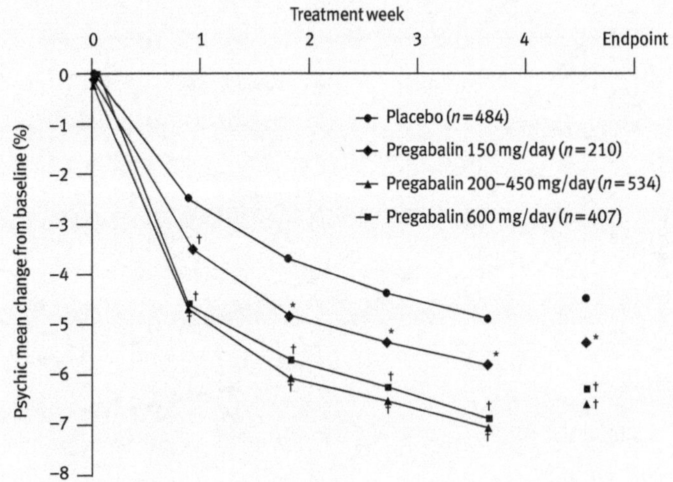

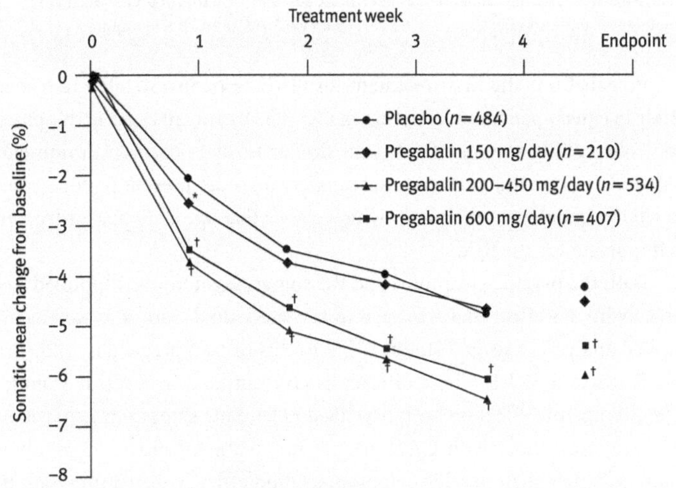

Figure 7.8 Pregabalin reduces both psychic and somatic symptoms of GAD: pooled analysis from six GAD studies. GAD, generalised anxiety disorder; LOCF, last observation carried forward; PBO, placebo; PGB, pregabalin; VEN, venalafaxine. **P*<0.05; †*P*<0.001 vs placebo; Endpoint: 4 weeks (LOCF). Six studies combined.

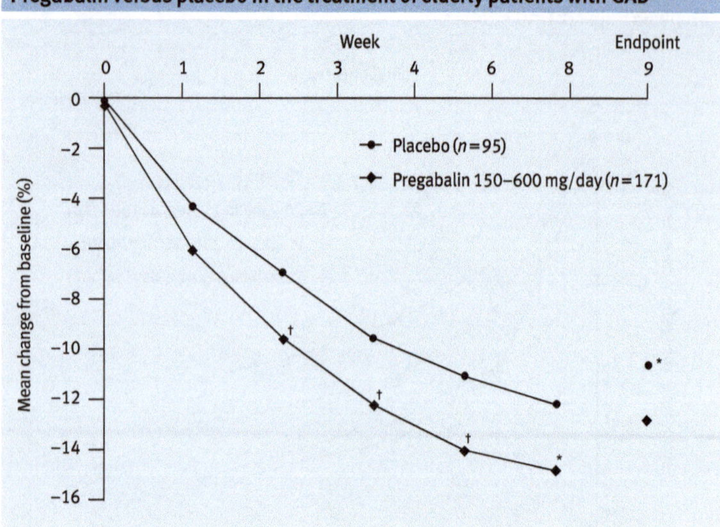

Figure 7.9 Pregabalin versus placebo in the treatment of elderly patients with GAD. GAD, generalised anxiety disorder. $^{*}P<0.05$, $^{\dagger}P<0.01$ vs placebo. Mean HAM-A baseline score was 26.5. An 8-week, double-blind, randomised placebo-controlled trial of pregabalin in the treatment of patients over the age of 65 years with GAD. Adapted from Montgomery et al.[41]

Pregabalin is the first treatment for GAD to be investigated in a specific study in elderly patients over the age of 65.[41] The treatment effect in this placebo-controlled study was significant and similar to that observed in non-elderly patients. GAD is the most common anxiety disorder presenting for treatment in elderly people and the result, which shows that age is no bar for treatment, is important for the field.

Both the psychic symptoms and the somatic symptoms responded well to pregabalin, an effect that was seen in the individual studies as well as in the pooled analysis of several studies.[69,78,81] In this respect pregabalin differs from the SSRIs and SNRIs where efficacy is concentrated on psychic symptoms. The therapeutic effect on both psychic and somatic symptoms is particularly relevant since those with GAD present for treatment most commonly with somatic rather than psychic symptoms. Good efficacy in treating both these sets of symptoms of GAD is important. A separate analysis of the effect of pregabalin on GI symptoms in the pooled analysis of six studies of GAD confirms this advantage.[82]

Sleep disturbance is a common presentation of GAD and is recognised as a core diagnostic symptom in DSM-IV. Pregabalin is effective and has a fast action in improving sleep disturbance compared with placebo in GAD, in contrast to SSRIs and SNRIs which tend to disrupt sleep.[81] An analysis of the effect of pregabalin on the depressive symptoms associated with GAD in one study[69] shows that both pregabalin and venlafaxine are effective compared with placebo and this benefit with pregabalin was also reported in the meta-analysis of six studies.[83] The frequently observed mild depressive symptoms appear to be part of GAD rather than representing a comorbid disorder. However, where MDD is present and the depressive symptoms reach a moderate or greater severity level then treatment with an antidepressant is indicated.

In summary, pregabalin is effective in GAD and has advantages not enjoyed by alternative treatments: it is fast in its action with differences from placebo significant by the fourth day.[70] It is effective in improving sleep and improving equally the psychic and somatic symptoms of GAD in contrast to SSRIs or SNRIs. It is effective in the treatment of pain and, as GAD is frequently comorbid with pain disorders and pain is a presenting symptom in as many as a third of GAD patients, this is a clear advantage, particularly when compared with SSRIs or benzodiazepines which are not thought to be effective in pain disorders. Pregabalin is clearly effective in short-term treatment but it is also effective compared with placebo in relapse prevention over a period of 6 months.[84]

Pregabalin is well tolerated with a level of adverse events comparable to that seen on placebo. The number of patients who discontinued treatment with pregabalin in the studies due to adverse events was small (11%), close to the number on placebo (9%), and compares very favourably with the 20% of patients who discontinued venlafaxine at the lowest dose, or 35% who discontinued lorazepam in the comparator studies. The most common adverse events are somnolence and dizziness which tend to improve with prolonged treatment. Unlike benzodiazepines pregabalin shows no signals of dependence either in animal models or in the extensive clinical trial programme. Discontinuation symptoms following abrupt termination of treatment do not appear to be a problem; the rate is low after both short-term and long-term treatment.

Benzodiazepines

Despite the acknowledged side effects and risks of dependence associated with benzodiazepines these drugs are still widely used in primary care in the treatment of GAD. To some extent this continued use is due to their long availability and hence familiarity. Their use also perhaps reflects a less than adequate assessment of the efficacy of benzodiazepines and the ratio of risk to benefit. The problem is compounded by the relatively weak evidence of efficacy accepted in the less demanding climate for testing efficacy in anxiety or anxiety neurosis, prevailing at the time that benzodiazepines were introduced, and by the failure to take into account the safety issues which, to be fair, became more evident over subsequent years. Studies that did not specify the nature of the anxiety disorder studied cannot provide evidence of efficacy in GAD; evidence can be obtained only from placebo-controlled studies that specifically studied GAD defined by accepted criteria.

There are suggestions that benzodiazepines may lose efficacy with time and this tolerance has been reported to lead to dose escalation and an increased risk of dependence. Benzodiazepines have profound effects on short-term memory, a property that has been found particularly useful in dental and surgical procedures where they are widely used for this purpose. The disturbances in cognition are also seen in the daytime even when taken at night, particularly with benzodiazepines that have a long half-life or when those with a short half-life are prescribed in the multiple daily dose regimens considered necessary in the treatment of daytime anxiety. Benzodiazepines are associated with daytime drowsiness which impairs the ability of the individual to work or function adequately and users should not drive or operate heavy machinery.

Concerns relating to tolerance, dose escalation and addiction[85,86] have led regulatory authorities in Europe to restrict the use of all benzodiazepines to short-term use for no longer than 3 months. This limits the suitability of benzodiazepines for the treatment of GAD which is a chronic disorder requiring treatment over long periods.

The evidence of the efficacy of benzodiazepines in GAD is modest and the number of placebo-controlled studies surprisingly small. In an early study in GAD defined using a short duration criterion, diazepam in a dose of 15 mg was shown to be significantly better than placebo over 8 weeks measured on the HAM-A.[87] Efficacy was greatest in the early weeks and then appeared to tail off. The question mark over the efficacy of the benzodiazepine in this study is also underlined by the greater treatment effect observed with imipramine in the same study. However, efficacy is reported for diazepam in several placebo-controlled studies.[87–92] A range of studies investigating 5-HT_3-receptor antagonists in GAD, which included diazepam as a reference anxiolytic drug and failed to separate from placebo, has regrettably never been properly published.[93] This leads to a very real concern that negative results often remain unpublished and that the efficacy of diazepam may not be strong.

The best evidence that benzodiazepines are effective in treating GAD defined by a longer duration comes from the placebo-controlled studies investigating the efficacy of pregabalin, in which benzodiazepines were included as reference agents. Lorazepam in a dose of 6 mg was effective at 4 weeks in two of the three studies.[80,81] At this high dose of lorazepam there were numerous dropouts (35%), higher than seen with pregabalin (11%) which was close to the placebo rate (9%). The therapeutic effect of lorazepam appeared early with a significant difference from placebo at 1 week observed with lorazepam, but only in one of the three studies, in contrast to pregabalin where a significant difference from placebo at 1 week was observed in all three lorazepam controlled studies and at all doses in the six pivotal placebo-controlled studies.[81]

The efficacy of alprazolam in GAD has been shown in a number of short-term placebo-controlled studies.[78,94,95] Alprazolam in a dose of 1.5 mg was the reference agent in a placebo-controlled study of the efficacy of three different doses of pregabalin.[78] Alprazolam and pregabalin showed a significantly greater reduction in HAM-A score compared with placebo at the endpoint of the 4-week study. Alprazolam separated significantly from placebo at one week measured on the HAM-A, as did the three doses of pregabalin. In this study therefore alprazolam was associated with early onset efficacy, though the treatment effect versus placebo at 1 week was about half that observed on all three doses of pregabalin.

In summary there is evidence that high doses of lorazepam 6 mg, diazepam 15 mg, and lower doses of high-potency benzodiazepines, eg alprazolam 1.5 mg, are effective in treating GAD, but the number of dropouts is high and the problem of impairment of cognition and concerns about the possible development of dependence, particularly over the medium and long term, limits their usefulness.

Buspirone

Buspirone, an azapirone drug that has partial agonist activity at the 5-HT_{1A} receptor, is one of the earlier medications that has shown efficacy in GAD although not all studies were positive. An early study in patients who would have fulfilled criteria for anxiety neurosis in the DSM version current at the time found similar efficacy between buspirone and diazepam.[96] Its efficacy in GAD as later defined is not well established and in one study it failed to show efficacy whereas venlafaxine was reported to be effective.[65] A meta-analysis of the studies carried out with buspirone concluded that the efficacy was comparable with that of benzodiazepines[97] but it is not generally a first choice treatment. Uncertainty about the therapeutic dose range and the appearance of unwanted effects such as dizziness attributable to the α-agonist actions of buspirone's active metabolite also detract from its value in treatment. There have been reports of a reduction in efficacy where buspirone follows treatment with benzodiazepines.

Forthcoming and other treatments for GAD

A number of treatments have been found to be effective in treating GAD judged by the criterion of at least one positive placebo-controlled study. These treatments would be expected sooner or later to join the small list of options approved for the treatment of GAD. To this could be added some treatments that have shown efficacy but may have been considered by the authorities to be lacking some component in the efficacy deemed necessary for licensing. Some are unlikely to be pursued because the treatments are now generic and the impetus to finance and conduct these studies is not forthcoming.

Quetiapine XR

This atypical antipsychotic has begun a comprehensive programme to investigate efficacy in both MDD and GAD. The MDD programme is complete and is currently under review by the various licensing agencies. Suffice to say there is clear efficacy in four out of five placebo-controlled studies in the acute treatment of MDD, including in elderly people, as well as in a long-term efficacy study.[98] Efficacy is seen in fixed doses of 50, 150 and 300 mg/day with an optimum ratio of efficacy to side effects at 150 mg/day. There is good evidence of fast onset of efficacy in MDD with separation from placebo consistently observed at 1 week and sustained to the end of the 6-week studies.

Some caution is needed in interpreting the results of the studies of quetiapine XR in GAD since these have not yet been published in peer-reviewed journals, although they have been presented at international conferences and can be checked on the AstraZeneca website (www.astrazenecaclinicaltrials.com). Two studies reported early and persistent efficacy of quetiapine XR in the short-term, 8-week treatment of GAD. In one study quetiapine in doses of 50 or 150 mg/day were significantly better than placebo at both 4 days and endpoint. In the other study quetiapine in doses of 150 or 300 mg were again effective at 4 days and endpoint. In both studies the 150 mg dose was significantly better than both placebo and the comparators in the two separate studies, paroxetine 20 mg and escitalopram 10 mg. The 150 mg dose of quetiapine was therefore the most effective dose with the most consistent efficacy on the secondary study measures.

Quetiapine XR appeared well tolerated with somnolence dizziness, and dry mouth being the most common adverse events. At the lower doses weight gain was minimal and the rate of extrapyramidal symptoms observed was less than that seen with duloxetine, the comparator used in the MDD study. Concerns about the metabolic syndrome have led the FDA not to approve the licence for monotherapy in GAD.

Agomelatine

Agomelatine is now licensed as an antidepressant in the EU and some other countries at doses of 25–50 mg/day. There is evidence of superior efficacy compared with venlafaxine and sertraline, driven to some degree by the much better tolerability and compliance observed with agomelatine. Because of its 5-HT2C-antagonist properties agomelatine does not increase serotonin or noradrenaline levels. Discontinuation symptoms are therefore not observed following abrupt cessation of treatment.[57] There are also low levels of sexual dysfunction or other well-known serotoninergic side effects. There are some concerns about possible liver toxicity, particularly at the higher dose, which requires monitoring.

In GAD there is one positive placebo-controlled study[99] in which agomelatine showed efficacy with a typical treatment effect and separation from placebo in the 12-week study (Figure 7.10). We await further studies.

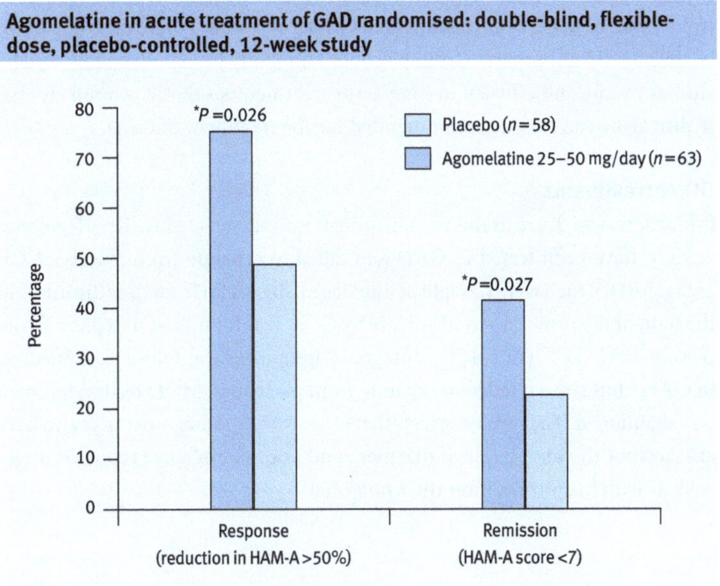

Figure 7.10 Agomelatine in acute treatment of GAD: randomised, double-blind, flexible-dose, placebo-controlled, 12-week study. GAD, generalised anxiety disorder; HAM-A, Hamilton Anxiety rating scale. Mean baseline HAM-A scores: placebo 28.6, agomelatine 29.0. Adapted from Stein et al.[99]

Imipramine

The efficacy in GAD of the tricyclic antidepressant (TCA), imipramine, was shown in an 8-week study compared with placebo in patients whose GAD symptoms had persisted for at least 4 months.[87] The study included the benzodiazepine diazepam as a comparator given at a high dose of 15 mg/day. The effect was largely confined to the psychic symptoms of anxiety in contrast to diazepam. Although diazepam was associated with efficacy early in the study at 2 weeks, by the end of the study imipramine showed a significant advantage over diazepam. Similar results are seen in the comparison with alprazolam.[100] The absence of long-term efficacy, regarded as mandatory in the EU, and the reported cardiotoxicity and poor tolerability of the TCAs have compromised the use of imipramine in GAD and it is unlikely that it will ever be licensed for GAD.

Hydroxazine

The antihistamine hydroxazine has been found to be effective in placebo-controlled studies in the acute treatment of GAD[101] in a study where the comparator buspirone did not separate from placebo. This study has not been followed by studies examining efficacy in long-term treatment so that it is unlikely that hydroxazine can ever be recommended for the treatment of GAD.

Other treatments

β-blockers, which are useful in managing tremor associated with performance anxiety, have been tested in GAD and failed to separate from placebo. CCK antagonists, which were thought at one stage to be useful in anxiety disorders in the light of the provocation of anxiety by CCK, was found not to separate from placebo in GAD.[102] The 5-HT_{1A}-antagonist ipsapirone was found to be effective in GAD[91] but since it failed to separate from placebo in MDD its development was abandoned. The result suggests that other 5-HT_{1A}-antagonist may also have efficacy but the high levels of dizziness and poor compliance reported might well, as with buspirone, limit their potential.

Chapter 8

Psychological treatment

Despite the body of evidence showing the disability associated with GAD there are still many who do not recognise that GAD is a serious, dangerous and impairing disorder and who prefer to believe that right living, right thinking and exercise are the answer. Formal investigation of the possible efficacy of these types of intervention has not been undertaken in adequately controlled trials that take account of confounding variables such as the halo effects of enthusiasts. In a climate of cost cutting there is a risk that alternative approaches such as self-help manuals, counselling and exercise are promoted in order to save money on drug budgets without appropriate critical reference to the quality of the evidence base.

The evidence supporting the efficacy of psychological treatments in GAD is derived from a small number of studies relative to the large body of evidence for the efficacy of pharmacological treatments. Nevertheless there is a growing literature on the use of behavioural therapies and several treatment packages have been proposed. These have included anxiety management through relaxation therapy, components of cognitive therapy aimed at addressing worrying and behavioural challenges to confront worry behaviours.[103,104]

The problem of identifying an adequate control treatment group in studies of psychological treatments makes for a major difficulty in obtaining a valid and reliable estimate of efficacy. Various designs have been applied, for example, taking a no treatment group as a control, or a group remaining on the waiting list for treatment, but these are flawed by the potential bias of untreated patients exaggerating their symptoms and those receiving treatment reporting responses that may be due to non-specific factors unrelated to the treatment. Giving or receiving a treatment perceived by both therapist and patient as effective carries an additional therapeutic effect over and above that which may be due to the treatment itself. It is not possible to control for this except by comparing treatments given under open conditions by doctors who believe in the efficacy of the comparator treatments. It is essential in these studies to use raters blinded to treatment to try to counter the bias of the therapist.

Some studies indicate that cognitive–behavioural therapy (CBT) and relaxation therapy produced a similar improvement in symptoms.[104,105] In a study where CBT was compared with anxiety management, despite the CBT group having greater contact, both treatments were similar in effect and superior to psychotherapy at 6 months. Direct comparisons of CBT with analytical psychotherapy have favoured CBT[106] which supports the generally held view that analytical psychotherapy is not helpful in GAD. Comparisons of CBT with behaviour therapy or a waiting list control have reported that most significant improvement is seen with CBT compared with the wait list control and that the therapeutic gains are maintained over the longer term.[104,105,107]

The comparisons of different psychological treatments suggest that CBT is an effective treatment for GAD. For a reliable assessment, however, one would wish that efficacy was supported with evidence from studies that had used more stringent methodology.

Psychological and psychopharmacological treatments

Assessing the efficacy of psychological treatment relative to pharmacotherapy is not easy on the basis of the studies that have been carried out in this area. For a fair comparison recognised pharmacological treatments for GAD, in doses with established efficacy, must be used. For example, a study that compared CBT, anxiety management and lorazepam given in a dose of 3 mg/day, then 2 mg/day followed by 1 mg/day, each for a period of 10 days, does not meet this standard. The drug produced an early response that tailed off during the study whereas the effect of psychological treatment appeared later but was sustained. Clearly no conclusions can be drawn from such a poor design.[108]

CBT is sometimes compared in an open treatment arm of a study where drug or placebo is given under double-blind conditions. In this type of design the CBT, which has the added effect of the reassurance of open treatment, cannot be fairly compared with the drug or placebo arms which lack this reassuring effect. The claim that CBT and CBT plus diazepam had greater efficacy than diazepam or placebo is thus overstated.[109] For a fair comparison between a pharmacological treatment and a psychological treatment, which is given openly with both the therapist and patient knowing that they are receiving what they consider an effective treatment, the pharmacological treatment also needs to be given openly. In this way the therapist and patient are reassured by knowing the treatment is active. Therapist contact time needs to be equalised between groups and improvement assessed by raters blind to the study.

Independent raters will, to some extent, reduce the bias of open studies though the patient is inevitably aware of the nature of the treatment. The bias of this knowledge and beliefs about the treatment, in addition to dependence on the therapist, may exaggerate response. Such a design, which might cope with the extra non-specific benefits that accompany open treatment, does not appear to have been attempted.

In studies investigating the efficacy of pharmacotherapy, recording of the discontinuations from treatment is mandatory and the analysis of efficacy is carried out in the randomised population on a last observation carried forward analysis to address the influence of early withdrawals. These data are rarely provided in studies of CBT. Ignoring the substantial number of patients who refuse treatment or discontinue early produces a biased sample that will distort the results in the direction of those who benefit from treatment.

Chapter 9

Which treatments, when and for how long?

The evidence base for the pharmacological treatment of GAD is now substantial. However, there are few studies comparing treatments to inform rational choices either for GAD as a whole or for selective treatments for particular subgroups of GAD. The best guidance therefore comes from a careful analysis of the data from placebo-controlled studies that indicate the strengths and weaknesses of particular treatments.

How long should treatment be continued?

A number of relapse prevention studies have demonstrated the benefits of long-term treatment. These studies are designed to investigate whether persistence of treatment in those who respond to short-term therapy will lead to fewer patients having exacerbations of symptoms or relapse than placebo. These studies usually run for some 6 months to a year after the acute treatment period is complete. The consistent results from these studies show that the risk of relapse is about three times higher in those treated with placebo than in those receiving active treatment for GAD, even over this relatively short period. This continued therapeutic and protective effect supports the recommendation that short-term prophylaxis is insufficient and that treatment should be continued to keep the individual well. The studies vary slightly in their design features and the differences observed between treatments in the significant benefit in long-term outcome compared with placebo probably arises from these variations in design rather than any inherent disparity in the efficacy of treatments. The relapse prevention studies have been carried out in patients with moderate-to-severe GAD and therefore in these patients treatment in the long term is indicated. In patients with severe or dysfunctional GAD there are reasonable grounds for continuing the treatment indefinitely.

There is no evidence of loss of efficacy in relapse prevention whether the randomisation to the continued drug or placebo occurs early or later in the course of treatment. Efficacy is not dependent on the total length of exposure to a treatment, whether 9 or 18 months. There is no evidence of loss of efficacy for any of the licensed treatments for GAD.

The recommendation of the British Association of Psychopharmacology[110] is that treatment should be continued for 6 months after a response to 12 weeks' treatment. In my view, this does not take adequate account of the probability that patients with GAD will remain well if treatment with medication is continued for longer periods.

The long-term efficacy of cognitive–behavioural therapy (CBT) is supported by a lower level of scientific evidence, being based on uncontrolled open studies. It is claimed that there are fewer relapses on CBT than with medication but the comparison is misleading, not least because the studies on CBT generally recruit less severe patients who do not have the same high relapse rates.

In those with moderate or severe GAD, if the treatment is discontinued, for whatever reason, there is likely to be a relapse over the subsequent months. The frequency of monitoring needs to be increased so that treatment, preferably having a fast onset of effect, can be initiated at the first signs of relapse. There are, as yet, too few data from long-term comparator studies to suggest that one effective licensed treatment for GAD is better than another. The doctor is free to choose the treatment that is best tolerated and which best suits the pattern of predominant complaints and comorbidity in the individual sufferer.

Choice of treatment based on predominant complaints or comorbidity

Somatic symptoms

Somatic symptoms are the most common complaint of those with GAD and there is a clear difference between the various treatments in their ability to improve these symptoms. In general the selective serotonin reuptake inhibitors (SSRIs) and serotonin noradrenaline reuptake inhibitors (SNRIs) are less effective in managing these symptoms. While they have some benefit this is often not evident in short-term studies where clear evidence of benefit on psychic symptoms is consistently observed. On the other hand somatic symptoms respond rapidly to pregabalin in doses of 200–600 mg/day which show a separation from placebo as early as day 4, with the benefit persisting to the end of the study. Pregabalin therefore should be considered early in these patients. The recommendation to use benzodiazepines to treat the somatic symptoms of GAD is not supported by the same strength of evidence and the risk–benefit assessment of using a potentially dependence-inducing treatment is negative.

Sleep disturbance

Sleep disturbance is a core diagnostic symptom of GAD and is reported as the main presenting complaint in some 35% of those with GAD attending primary care. SSRIs and SNRIs are often disruptive on sleep particularly in the early stages of treatment. Duloxetine and sertraline are particularly troublesome. For this reason SSRIs and SNRIs are not the preferred choice for those with predominant sleep problems. Pregabalin by contrast has a beneficial effect on sleep disturbance which is seen early and persists and pregabalin should be considered a priority in those with prominent sleep difficulties.

Depression

Major depressive disorder (MDD) is one of the most frequent comorbid conditions in GAD and for patients with both GAD and MDD it makes sense to select a treatment that is effective in both. Since both the SSRIs and the SNRIs have shown efficacy in both MDD and GAD they are obvous first-line treatments where there is overlap. Anxiety symptoms subside when the MDD is treated with SSRIs or SNRIs and depressive symptoms when the GAD is treated. Prospective trials of efficacy in GAD comorbid with MDD would be helpful. In GAD with mild depression that does not meet the diagnostic criteria for MDD there appears to be no advantage for antidepressants compared with other treatments. Pregabalin and venlafaxine were equally effective in GAD compared with placebo in improving mild depressive symptoms as measured on the Hamilton Depression Scale (HAMD)[111] and it seems likely that these mild symptoms are part of GAD rather than representing a comorbid depressive disorder. Benzodiazepines are thought to be ineffective or even to make depression worse and, since they are not licensed for either GAD or depression and have other well-known risks, they should be avoided.

GAD and bipolar depression

There is a high level of comorbidity between GAD and bipolar disorder and treating GAD under these circumstances is particularly difficult. It is recommended that antidepressants in general should be avoided in bipolar depression as they may cause switches to mania and are not particularly effective. Lithium, which is widely used, has been shown to be effective in mania but is less effective for depression and in recent studies in bipolar depression lithium did not separate from placebo in the short or long term.[112] The only treatment licensed in bipolar depression in the EU is quetiapine and some very recent data show placebo-controlled efficacy of this drug at relatively low doses in both GAD and MDD. The use of a licensed treatment for GAD concomitantly with a licensed treatment for bipolar depression would appear to be the only evidence-based option.

GAD in elderly people

The treatment of GAD in elderly people has not, until recently, been well investigated. This is regrettable since GAD is the most frequent anxiety diagnosis in elderly patients attending for treatment and is therefore a large public health issue. It is reported that about half of the elderly population with GAD have a recent onset.[113] Post-hoc meta-analyses of placebo-controlled datasets suggest that some treatments for GAD appear to be effective in older patients aged 60–65 as well as younger patients.[114,115] A small placebo-controlled study looking at anxiety disorders, including GAD, in elderly people showed benefit with citalopram; however, given that there were no other placebo-controlled data on the efficacy of citalopram in GAD this finding is of limited value.[116] Pregabalin in a flexible dose has been shown to be effective compared with placebo and well tolerated in a specific study of GAD in patients over the age of 65.[41] The treatment effect was similar to that observed in non-elderly GAD suffers and there appeared to be no diminution of treatment effect in the smaller subgroups over the age of 70 or 75.[41] Until further studies become available pregabalin has the most secure evidence base for the treatment of GAD in elderly people.

References

1. APA. Diagnostic and Statistical Manual of Mental Disorders (DSM-IIIR). 3rd edn. Washington: American Psychiatric Association, 1987.
2. APA. Diagnostic and Statistical Manual of Mental Disorders (DSM-III). Washington: American Psychiatric Association, 1980.
3. APA. Diagnostic and Statistical Manual of Mental Disorders (DSM-IV). Washington: American Psychiatric Association, 1994.
4. APA. Diagnostic Criteria from DSM-IV-TR. Washington: American Psychiatric Association, 2000.
5. APA. Diagnostic and Statistical Manual of Mental Disorders (DSM-II). Washington: American Psychiatric Association, 1968.
6. APA. Diagnostic and Statistical Manual of Mental Disorders. Washington: American Psychiatric Association, 1952.
7. Pecknold JC, Matas M, Howarth BG, et al. Evaluation of buspirone as an antianxiety agent: buspirone and diazepam versus placebo. Can J Psychiatry 1989; 34:766–71.
8. Bohm C, Placchi M, Stallone F, et al. A double-blind comparison of buspirone, clobazam, and placebo in patients with anxiety treated in a general practice setting. J Clin Psychopharmacol 1990;10:38S–42S.
9. Hamilton M. The assessment of anxiety states by rating. Br J Med Psychol 1959;32:50–5.
10. Angst J, Gamma A, Baldwin DS, et al. The generalized anxiety spectrum: prevalence, onset, course and outcome. Eur Arch Psychiatry Clin Neurosci 2009; 259:37–45.
11. WHO. International Classification of Diseases 10th revision (ICD-10). Geneva: World Health Organization, 1992.
12. Wittchen H-U, Jacobi F. Size and burden of mental disorders in Europe – a critical review and appraisal of 27 studies. Eur Neuropsychopharmacol 2005; 15:357–76.
13. Wittchen H-U, Kessler RC, Beesdo K, et al. Generalized anxiety and depression in primary care: prevalence, recognition, and management. J Clin Psychiatry 2002; 63(Suppl 8):24–34.
14. Kessler RC, Wittchen H-U. Patterns and correlates of generalized anxiety disorder in community samples. J Clin Psychiatry 2002; 63(Suppl 8):4–10.
15. Carter RM, Wittchen H-U, Pfister H, et al. One-year prevalence of subthreshold and threshold DSM-IV generalized anxiety disorder in a nationally representative sample. Depress Anxiety 2001; 13:78–88.
16. Beekman AT, de Beurs E, van Balkom AJ, et al. Anxiety and depression in later life: Co-occurrence and communality of risk factors. Am J Psychiatry 2000; 157:89–95.
17. Baldwin DS, Huusom AK, Maehlum E. Escitalopram and paroxetine in the treatment of generalised anxiety: randomized, placebo-controlled, double-blind study. Br J Psychiatry 2006; 189:264–72.
18. Allgulander C, Dahl AA, Austin C, et al. Efficacy of sertraline in a 12-week trial for generalized anxiety disorder. Am J Psychiatry 2004; 161:1642–49.

19. Keller M. Raising the expectations of long-term treatment strategies in anxiety disorders. Psychopharm Bull 2002; 36(Suppl 2):166–74.
20. Schoevers RA, Deeg DJ, van Tilburg W, et al. Depression and generalized anxiety disorder: co-occurrence and longitudinal patterns in elderly patients. Am J Geriatr Psychiatry 2005; 13:31–9.
21. Olsson I, Mykletun A, Dahl AA. Recognition and treatment recommendations for generalized anxiety disorder and major depressive episode: a cross-secional study among general practitioners in Norway. Primary Care Companion to J Clin Psychiatry 2006; 8:340–7.
22. Andrews G, Sanderson K, Sluys M, et al. Why does the burden of disease persist? Relating the burdenof anxiety and depression to effectiveness of treatment. Bull World Health Organ 2000; 78:446–54.
23. Maier W, Falkai P. The epidemiology of comorbidity between depression, anxiety disorders and somatic diseases. Int Clin Psychopharmacol 1999; 14:1–6.
24. Wulsin LR, Arnold LM, Hillard JR. Axis I disorders in ER patients with atypical chest pain. Int J Psychiatry Med 1991; 21:37–46.
25. Kane FJ, Harper RG, Wittels E. Angina as a symptom of psychiatric illness. South Med J 1988; 11:1412–6.
26. Wittchen H-U, Zhao S, Kessler RC, et al. DSMIII-R generalized anxiety disorder in the national comorbidity survey. Arch Gen Psychiatry 1994; 51:355–64.
27. Alonso J, Angermeyer MC, ESEMeD/MHEDEA 2000 Investigators. 12-Month comorbidity patterns and associated factors in Europe: results from the European Study of the Epidemiology of Mental Disorders (ESEMeD) project. Acta Psychiatr Scand 2004; 109(Suppl 420):28–37.
28. Angst J, Vollrath M. The natural history of anxiety disorders. Acta Psychiatr Scand 1991; 446–52.
29. Marcuso DM, Townsend MH, Mercante DE. Long-term follow-up of generalized anxiety disorder. Compr Psychiatry 1993; 34:441–6.
30. Souery D, Oswald P, Massat I, et al. Clinical factors associated with treatment resistance in major depressive disorder: results from a European multicenter study. J Clin Psychiatry. 2007; 68:1062–70.
31. Judd LL, Kessler RC, Paulus MP, et al. Comorbidity as a fundamental feature of generalized anxiety disorders: results from the National Comorbidity Study (NCS). Acta Psychiatr Scand Suppl 1998; 393:6–11.
32. Üstün TB, Sartorius N. Mental Illness in General Health Care. Chichester: John Wiley, 1995.
33. Angst J, Gamma A, Bienvenu J, et al. Varying temporal criteria for generalized anxiety disorder: prevalence and clinical characteristics in a young cohort. Psychol Med 2006; 36:1283–92.
34. Kroenke K, Spitzer RL, Williams JB, et al. Anxiety disorders in primary care: prevalence, impairment, comorbidity, and detection. Ann Intern Med 2007; 146:317–25.
35. Schonfeld WH, Verboncoeur CJ, Fifer SK, et al. The functioning and well-being of patients with unrecognized anxiety disorders and major depressive disorder. J Affect Disord 1997; 43:105–19.
36. Jones GN, Ames SC, Jeffries SK, et al. Utilization of medical services and quality of life among low-income patients with generalized anxiety disorder attending primary care clinics. Int J Psychiatry Med 2001; 31:183–98.
37. Kessler RC, DuPont RL, Berglund P, et al. Impairment in pure and comorbid generalized anxiety disorder and major depression at 12 months in two national surveys. Am J Psychiatry 1999; 156:1915–23.
38. Wittchen H-U, Carter RM, Pfister H, et al. Disabilities and quality of life in pure and comorbid generalized anxiety disorder and major depression in a national survey. Int Clin Psychopharmacol 2000; 15:319–28.

39. Boyer P, Mahe VV, Hackett D. Social adjustment in generalised anxiety disorder: a long-term placebo-controlled study of venlafaxine extended release. Eur Psychiatry 2004;19:272–9.
40. Grant BF, Hasin DS, Stinson FS, et al. Prevalence, correlates, comorbidity, and compariative disability of DSM IV generalized anxiety disorder in the USA: results from the National Epidemiologic Survey on alcohol and related conditions. Psychol Med 2005; 35:1747–59.
41. Montgomery S, Chatamra K, Pauer L, et al. Efficacy and safety of pregabalin in elderly people with generalised anxiety disorder. Br J Psychiatry 2008; 193:389–94.
42. Hunt C, Issakidis C, Andrews G. DSMIV generalized anxiety disorder in the Australian National Survey of mental health and well-being. Psychol Med 2002; 32:649–59.
43. Olfson M, Gameroff MJ. Generalized anxiety disorder, somatic pain and health care costs. Gen Hosp Psychiatry 2007; 29:310–6.
44. Souetre E, Lozet H, Cimarosti I, et al. Cost of anxiety disorders: impact of comorbidity. J Psychosom Res 1994; 38:151–60.
45. Roy-Byrne P, Wagner A. Primary care perspectives on generalized anxiety disorder. J Clin Psychiatry 2000; 65; Suppl 13:20–6.
46. Wittchen H-U, Nelson CB, Lachner G. Prevalence of mental disorders and psychosocial impairments in adolescents and young adults. Psychol Med 1998; 28:109–26.
47. Zigmond AS, Snaith RP. The hospital anxiety and depression scale. Acta Psychiatr Scand 1983; 67:361–70.
48. Lipman RS, Covi L, Rickels K, et al. Selected measures in outpatient evaluation. In: Efron DH (ed.) Psychopharmacology: a review of progress. Washington: US Government Printing Office, 1968:249–54.
49. Raskin A, Schulterbrandt J, Reatig N, et al. Replication of factors of psychopathology in interview, ward behavior and self-report ratings of hospitalized depressives. J Nerv Ment Dis 1969; 148:87–98.
50. Guy W. ECDEU Assessment Manual for Psychopharmacology. Rockville, MD: National Institute of Mental Health, 1976:218–22.
51. Sheehan KH, Sheehan DV. Assessing treatment effects in clinical trials with the Discan metric of the Sheehan Disability Scale. Int Clin Psychopharmacol 2008; 23:70–83.
52. Kennedy SH, Andersen HF, Lam RW. Efficacy of escitalopram in the treatment of major depressive disorder compared with conventional selective serotonin reuptake inhibitors and venlafaxine XR: a meta-analysis. J Psychiatry Neurosci 2006; 31:122–31.
53. Montgomery SA, Baldwin DS, Blier P, et al. Which antidepressants have demonstrated superior efficacy? A review of the evidence. Int Clin Psychopharmacol 2007; 22:323–29.
54. Pollack MH, Zaninelli R, Goddard A, et al. Paroxetine in the treatment of generalized anxiety disorder: a placebo-controlled, flexible-dosage trial. J Clin Psychiatry 2001; 62:350–7.
55. Rickels K, Zaninelli R, McCafferty J, et al. Paroxetine treatment of generalized anxiety disorder: a double-blind, placebo-controlled study. Am J Psychiatry 2003; 160:749–56.
56. Stocchi F, Nordera G, Jokinen RH, et al. Efficacy and tolerability of paroxetine for the long-term treatment of generalized anxiety disorder. J Clin Psychiatry 2003; 64:250–8.
57. Montgomery SA, Kennedy SH, Burrows GD, et al. Absence of discontinuation symptoms with agomelatine and occurrence of discontinuation symptoms with paroxetine: a randomized, double-blind, placebo-controlled discontinuation study. Int Clin Psychopharmacol 2004; 19:271–80.
58. Baldwin DS, Montgomery SA, Nil R, et al. Discontinuation symptoms in depression and anxiety disorders. Int J Neuropsychopharmacol 2007; 10:84.
59. Davidson JR, Bose A, Korotzer A, et al. Escitalopram in the treatment of generalized anxiety disorder: double-blind, placebo controlled, flexible-dose study. Depress Anxiety 2004; 19:234–40.

60. Goodman WK, Bose A, Wang Q. Treatment of generalized anxiety disorder with escitalopram: pooled results from double-blind, placebo-controlled trials. J Affect Disord 2005; 87:161–7.
61. Allgulander C, Florea I, Huusom AK. Prevention of relapse in generalized anxiety disorder by escitalopram treatment. Int J Neuropsychopharmacol 2006; 5:495–505.
62. Brawman-Mintzer O, Knapp R, Rynn M, et al. Sertraline treatment for Generalized Anxiety Disorder: a randomized, double-blind, placebo-controlled study. J Clin Psychiatry 2006; 67:874–81.
63. Rynn MA, Siqueland L, Rickels K. Placebo-controlled trial of sertraline in the treatment of children with generalized anxiety disorder. Am J Psychiatry 2001; 158:2008–14.
64. Rickels K, Pollack MH, Sheehan DV, et al. Efficacy of extended-release venlafaxine in nondepressed outpatients with generalized anxiety disorder. Am J Psychiatry 2000; 157:968–74.
65. Davidson JR, DuPont RL, Hedges D, et al. Efficacy, safety, and tolerability of venlafaxine extended release and buspirone in outpatients with generalized anxiety disorder. J Clin Psychiatry 1999; 60:528–35.
66. Gelenberg AJ, Lydiard RB, Rudolph RL, et al. Efficacy of venlafaxine extended-release capsules in nondepressed outpatients with generalized anxiety disorder: a 6-month randomized controlled trial. J Am Med Assoc 2000; 283:3082–8.
67. Allgulander C, Hackett D, Salinas E. Venlafaxine extended release (ER) in the treatment of generalised anxiety disorder: twenty-four-week placebo-controlled dose response study. Br J Psychiatry 2001; 179:15–22.
68. Montgomery SA, Sheehan DV, Meoni P, et al. Characterization of the longitudinal course of improvement in generalized anxiety disorder during long-term treatment with venlafaxine XR. J Psychiatr Res 2002; 36:209–17.
69. Montgomery SA, Tobias K, Zornberg GL, et al. Efficacy and safety of pregabalin in the treatment of generalized anxiety disorder: a 6-week, multicenter, randomized, double-blind, placebo-controlled comparison of pregabalin and venlafaxine. J Clin Psychiatry 2006; 67:771–82.
70. Kasper S, Berman B, Nivoli G, et al. Efficacy of pregabalin and venlafaxine XR in Generalized Disorder: results of a double-blind, placebo-controlled 8-week trial. Int Clin Psychopharmacol 2009; In press.
71. Lenox-Smith AJ, Reynolds A. A double-blind, randomised, placebo controlled study of venlafaxine XL in patients with generalised anxiety disorder in pirmary care. Br J Gen Pract 2003; 772–7.
72. Rynn MA, Riddle MA, Yeung PP, et al. Efficacy and safety of extended-release venlafaxine in the treatment of Generalized Anxiety Disorder in children and adolescents: two placebo-controlled trials. Am J Psychiatry 2007; 164:290–300.
73. Koponen H, Allgulander C, Erickson J, et al. Efficacy of duloxetine for the treatment of generalized anxiety disorder: implications for primary care physicians. Primary Care Companion J Clin Psychiatry 2007; 9:100–7.
74. Rynn M, Russell J, Erickson J, et al. Efficacy and safety of duloxetine in the treatment of generalized anxiety disorder: a flexible-dose, progressive-titration, placebo-controlled trial. Depress Anxiety 2008; 25:182–9.
75. Hartford J, Kornstein S, Liebowitz M, et al. Duloxetine as an SNRI treatment for generalized anxiety disorder: results from a placebo and active-controlled trial. Int Clin Psychopharmacol 2007; 22:167–74.
76. Dworkin RH, Corbin AE, Young JP Jr, et al. Pregabalin for the treatment of postherpetic neuralgia: a randomized, placebo-controlled trial. Neurology 2003; 60:1274–83.
77. French JA, Kugler AR, Robbins JL, et al. Dose-response trial of pregabalin adjunctive therapy in patients with partial seizures. Neurology 2003; 60:1631–7.
78. Rickels K, Pollack MH, Feltner DE, et al. Pregabalin for treatment of generalized anxiety disorder: a 4-week, multicenter, double-blind, placebo-controlled trial of pregabalin and alprazolam. Arch Gen Psychiatry 2005; 62:1022–30.

79. Pohl RB, Feltner DE, Fieve RR, et al. Efficacy of pregabalin in the treatment of generalized anxiety disorder: double-blind, placebo-controlled comparison of BID versus TID dosing. J Clin Psychopharmacol 2005; 25:151–8.
80. Pande AC, Crockatt JG, Feltner DE, et al. Pregabalin in generalized anxiety disorder: a placebo-controlled trial. Am J Psychiatry 2003; 160:533–40.
81. Montgomery SA. Pregabalin for the treatment of generalised anxiety disorder. Expert Opin Pharmacother 2006; 7:2139–54.
82. Stein D J, Lydiard RB, Herman BK, et al. Impact of gastrointestinal symptoms on response to pregabalin in generalized anxiety disorder: results of a 6-study combined analysis. Int Clin Psychopharmacol 2009; In press.
83. Stein DJ, Baldwin DS, Baldinetti F, et al. Efficacy of pregabalin in depressive symptoms associated with generalied anxiety disorder: A pooled analysis of 6 studies. Eur Neuropsychopharmacol 2008; 18:422–30.
84. Feltner D, Wittchen H-U, Kavoussi R, et al. Long-term efficacy of pregabalin in generalized anxiety disorder. Int Clin Psychopharmacol 2008; 23:18–28.
85. Montgomery SA, Tyrer PJ. Benzodiazepines: time to withdraw. J R Coll Gen Pract 1988; 146–147.
86. Woods JH, Katz JL, Winger G. Benzodiazepines: use, abuse, and consequences. Pharmacol Rev 1992; 44:151–347.
87. Rickels K, Downing R, Schweizer E, et al. Antidepressants for the treatment of generalized anxiety disorder, a placebo-controlled comparison of imipramine, trazodone, and diazepam. Arch Gen Psychiatry 1993; 50:884–95.
88. Rickels K, Schweizer E, DeMartinis NA, et al. Gepirone and diazepam in generalized anxiety disorder: a placebo-controlled trial. J Clin Psychopharmacol 1997; 17:272–7.
89. Rickels K, DeMartinis NA, Aufdembrinke B. A double-blind, placebo-controlled trial of abecarnil and diazepam in the treatment of patients with generalized anxiety disorder. J Clin Psychopharmacol 2000; 20:12–8.
90. Ansseau M, Olié JP. Controlled comparison of the efficacy and safety of four doses of suriclone, diazepam, and placebo in generalized anxiety disorder. Psychopharmacology. 1991; 104:439–43.
91. Boyer WF, Feighner JP. A placebo-controlled double-blind multicenter trial of two doses of ipsapirone versus diazepam in generalized anxiety disorder. Int Clin Psychopharmacol 1993; 8:173–6.
92. Fontaine R, Annable L, Chouinard G, et al. Bromazepam and diazepam in generalized anxiety : a placebo-controlled study with measurement of drug plasma concentrations. J Clin Psychopharmacol 1983; 3: 80–7.
93. Freeman AM III, Westphal JR, Norris GT, et al. Efficacy of ondansetron in the treatment of generalized anxiety disorder. Depress Anxiety 1997; 5:140–1.
94. Lydiard RB, Ballenger JC, Rickels K. A double-blind evaluation of the safety and efficacy of abecarnil, alprazolam, and placebo in outpatients with generalized axiety disorder. Abecarnil Work Group. J Clin Psychiatry 1997; 58:11–8.
95. Moller HJ, Volz HP, Reimann IW, et al. Opipramol for the treatment of generalized anxiety disorder: a placebo-controlled trial including an alprazolam-treated group. J Clin Psychopharmacol 2001; 21:59–65.
96. Goldberg HL, Finnerty RJ. The comparative efficacy of buspirone and diazepam in the treatment of anxiety. Am J Psychiatry 1979; 136:1184–7.
97. Gammans RE, Stringfellow JC, Hvizdos AJ, et al. Use of buspirone in patients with generalized anxiety disorder and coexisting depressive symptoms. A meta-analysis of eight randomised controlled studies. Neuropsychobiology 1992; 25:193–201.
98. Montgomery SA. Clinically relevant outcome measures in MDD: focus on the latest quetiapine XR data. Presented at: 8th International Forum on Mood and Anxiety Disorders, Vienna, Austria; November 12–14, 2008; SO 0401.

99. Stein DJ, Ahokas AA, de Bodinat C. Efficacy of agomelatine in generalized anxiety disorder: a randomized, double-blind, placebo-controlled study. J Clin Psychopharmacol 2008; 28:561–6.
100. Hoehn-Saric R, McLeod DR, Zimmerli WD. Differential effects of alprazolam and imipramine in generalized anxiety disorder: somatic versus psychic symptoms. J Clin Psychiatry. 1988; 49:293–301.
101. Lader M, Scotto JC. A multicentre double-blind comparison of hydroxysine, buspirone and placebo in patients with generalized anxiety disorder. Psychopharmacology (Berlin). 1998; 139:402–6.
102. Adams JB, Pyke RE, Costa J, et al. A double-blind, placebo-controlled study of a CCK-B receptor antagonist, CI-988, in patients with generalized anxiety disorder. J Clin Psychopharmacol 1995; 15:428–34.
103. Brown TA, O'Leary TA, Barlow DH. Generalized anxiety dDisorder. In: Barlow DH, ed. Clinical Handbook of Psychological Disorders. New York: Guilford Press, 1993:137–88.
104. Borkovec TD, Costello E. Efficacy of applied relaxation and cognitive-behavioral therapy in the treatment of generalized anxiety disorder. J Consult Clin Psychol 1993; 61:611–9.
105. Barlow DH, Rapee RM, Brown TA. Behavioral treatment of generalized anxiety disorder. Behav Ther 1992; 23:551–70.
106. Durham RC, Murphy T, Allan T, et al. Cognitive therapy, analytic psychotherapy and anxiety management training for generalised anxiety disorder. Br J Psychiatry. 1994; 165:315–23.
107. Durham RC, Turvey AA. Cognitive therapy vs behaviour therapy in the treatment of chronic general anxiety. Behav Res Ther 1987; 25:229–34.
108. Lindsay WR, Gamsu CV, McLaughlin E, et al. A controlled trial of treatments for generalized anxiety. Br J Clin Psychol 1987; 26:3–15.
109. Power KG, Simpson RJ, Swanson V, et al. A controlled comparison of cognitive-behavior therapy, diazepam, and placebo in the management of generalized anxiety. J Anxiety Disord 1990; 4:267–92.
110. Baldwin D, Anderson IM, Nutt D, et al. Evidence-based guidelines for the pharmacological treatment of anxiety disorders: recommendations from the British Association for Psychopharmacology. J Psychopharmacol 2005; 19:567–96.
111. Hamilton M. Development of rating scale for primary depressive illness. Br J Soc Clin Psychol 1967; 6:278–96.
112. Bowden CL, Calabrese JR, Sachs G, et al. A placebo-controlled 18-month trial of lamotrigine and lithium maintenance treatment in recently manic or hypomanic patients with bipolar I disorder. Arch Gen Psychiatry 2003; 60:392–400.
113. Blazer DG, Hughes D, George LK, et al. Generalized anxiety disorder. In: Robins LN, Regier DA (eds.) Psychiatric Disorders in America: the Epidemiologic Catchment Area Study. New York: The Free Press; 1991:180–203.
114. Katz IR, Reynolds CF, Alexopoulos GS, et al. Venlafaxine ER as a treatment for generalized anxiety disorder in older adults: pooled analysis of five randomized placebo-controlled clinical trials. J Am Geriatr Soc 2002; 50:18–25.
115. Davidson J, Allgulander C, Pollack MH, et al. Efficacy and tolerability of duloxetine in elderly patients with generalized anxiety disordr: a pooled analysis of four randomized, double-blind, placebo-controlled studies. Hum Psychopharmacol 2008; 23:519–26.
116. Lenze EJ, Mulsant BH, Shear MK, et al. Efficacy and tolerability of citalopram in the tretment of late-life anxiety disorders: results from an 8-week randomized, placebo-controlled trial. Am J Psychiatry 2005; 162:146–50.

Index compiled by Indexing Specialists (UK) Ltd
www.indexing.co.uk

Index